Root Operations:
Key to Procedure Coding in ICD-10-PCS

Ann Zeisset, RHIT, CCS, CCS-P
Ann Barta, MSA, RHIA

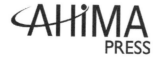

AHiMA
PRESS

ISBN: 978-1-58426-266-4
AHIMA Product No.: AC211010

AHIMA Staff:
Claire Blondeau, MBA, Senior Editor
Katie Greenock, Editorial and Production Coordinator
Ashley Sullivan, Assistant Editor
Ken Zielske, Director of Publications

All information contained within this book, including Web sites and regulatory information, was current and valid as of the date of publication. However, Web page addresses and the information on them may change or disappear at any time and for any number of reasons. The user is encouraged to perform his or her own general Web searches to locate any site addresses listed here that are no longer valid.

This publication is designed to provide accurate and authoritative information in regard to the subject matter covered. It is sold with the understanding that the publisher is not engaged in rendering legal, accounting, or other professional services. If legal advice or other expert assistance is required, the services of a competent professional person should be sought.

American Health Information Management Association
233 North Michigan Avenue, 21st Floor
Chicago, Illinois 60601-5809
ahima.org

Contents

About the Authors

Ann Zeisset, RHIT, CCS, CCS-P, is Manager of Professional Practice Resources for AHIMA. In this role, Zeisset provides professional expertise to AHIMA members, the media, and outside organizations on coding practice issues. She also authors and supports AHIMA online coding education, including the Coding Basics program; and is a technical advisor on ICD-9-CM, CPT, and ICD-10-CM/PCS coding publications. Zeisset has also authored many publications, including several on ICD-10-CM/PCS.

Prior to joining AHIMA in 1999, Zeisset served as director of Health Information/Utilization Management. Before that, Zeisset served in various coding roles, and has been an educator of coding and health information management (HIM) for more than 20 years at multiple colleges, and currently serves as adjunct faculty in the HIM Program at the University of Cincinnati. Zeisset has authored many coding-related articles, and has presented numerous seminars and educational sessions on coding and other HIM topics throughout the United States, including many for home health professionals. Zeisset recently completed a one-year contract between the Foundation for Research and Education (FORE) and CMS to determine potential impacts to CMS when converting from the ICD-9-CM coding system to the ICD-10-CM/PCS coding systems. Zeisset is a frequent author and speaker on ICD-10-CM/PCS, and serves as author and faculty for the AHIMA ICD-10-CM/PCS Academies to train trainers.

Zeisset was awarded the Distinguished Member award from the Southern Illinois Health Information Management Association (SILHIMA) in 2003 and the Certified Coding Specialist award in 2005; and the Professional Achievement award from the Illinois

Health Information Management Association (ILHIMA) in 2010. Zeisset received a bachelor's degree in organizational leadership at Greenville College in Greenville, Illinois.

Ann Barta, MSA, RHIA, AHIMA Professional Practice Resources Specialist, provides professional expertise on ICD-10 issues to AHIMA members, the media, and outside organizations. She is responsible for the development and presentation of educational materials on ICD-10-CM/PCS. In addition, she authors materials for and supports AHIMA online coding education, publications, and other products related to ICD-10-CM/PCS. Barta also served as faculty for the AHIMA ICD-10-CM/PCS Academies in 2009 and 2010.

Prior to joining AHIMA in September 2008, Barta participated in a one-year contract between the Foundation for Research and Education (FORE) and CMS to determine potential impacts to CMS when converting from the ICD-9-CM coding system to the ICD-10-CM/PCS coding systems. Prior to that, Barta served as a corporate coding manager for a large healthcare system. She has more than 30 years experience as an HIM director and coding consultant. She has been an educator of coding and HIM courses for more than 15 years, served as an Associate Dean for Health Sciences, and was System Coordinator for an RHIT program.

As an AHIMA member, Barta participates in various leadership positions, including serving on several RHIT Program Advisory Boards. Additionally, she was actively involved with the Illinois Health Information Management Association (ILHIMA), served on the Education Committee, and was a state coding instructor with the implementation of ICD-9-CM. Barta received a bachelor of science degree in medical records administration from Illinois State University in Normal, Illinois, and a master of Science in health services administration from Central Michigan University in Mt. Pleasant, Michigan.

About the Contributors

Melanie Endicott, MBA/HCM, RHIA, CCS, CCS-P, is a Practice Resources Specialist at AHIMA. In this role, she provides professional practice support for products and services related to coding and reimbursement, including seminars, publications, and Web-based training content and development. Endicott's primary focus at AHIMA is the development, maintenance, and delivery of the online Coding Basics program.

Endicott is also the program director of the health information technology (HIT) program at Spokane Community College in Spokane, Washington, and is an adjunct professor in the health information administration (HIA) program at Stephens College in Columbia, Missouri. Prior to her career as an educator and a member of the AHIMA staff, Melanie worked in a large acute care hospital performing both inpatient and outpatient coding and abstracting.

Endicott received her bachelor's degree in HIM in 1999 from Carroll College, in Helena, Montana, and her master's in business administration and health care management in 2005 from the University of Phoenix. During the past 10 years, she has been actively involved in local and state HIM activities by serving on multiple committees, and has held various officer positions. Endicott is also an AHIMA-Approved ICD-10-CM/PCS Trainer.

Kathy Giannangelo, MA, RHIA, CCS, CPHIMS, FAHIMA, has a comprehensive background in the field of clinical terminologies, classification, and data standards, with more than 30 years of experience in the health information management (HIM) field. In her current position as Director of Content Management for Apelon, Inc., she oversees the terminologies found within the core content suite, assists with the design and development of data sets and subsets to meet specific customer needs, and helps clients define terminology requirements, create or extend structured terminologies, and integrate terminology components into their products.

Previously she was a medical informaticist with Language and Computing (L&C), Inc., where her role was to support the ontology, modeling, sales, and product development activities related to the creation and implementation of natural language processing applications where clinical terminology and classification systems are used. Prior to L&C, she was a Director of Practice Leadership with AHIMA. Giannangelo has also served as senior nosologist for a health information services company and worked in various HIM roles including: vice president of product development, education specialist, director of medical records, quality assurance coordinator, and manager of a Centers for Disease Control and Prevention (CDC) research team. Giannangelo has developed classification, grouping, and reimbursement systems products for healthcare providers; conducted seminars; and provided consulting assessments throughout the United States, as well as in Canada, Australia, the United Kingdom, Ireland, and Bulgaria. In addition, she has authored numerous articles and created online continuing education courses on clinical terminologies. As adjunct faculty at the College of St. Scholastica, in Duluth, Minnesota, she teaches the graduate-level Clinical Vocabularies and Classification Systems course. In addition, she is actively involved as a volunteer in the HIM profession at the international, national, state, and local levels. Giannangelo holds a master's degree in HIM from the College of St. Scholastica.

Preface

On January 16, 2009, the U.S. Department of Health and Human Services (HHS) published a Final Rule for the adoption of ICD-10-CM and ICD-10-PCS code sets to replace the ICD-9-CM code set under rules, 45 CFR Parts 160 and 162 of the Health Insurance Portability and Accountability Act of 1996 (HIPAA). The compliance date for the two classification systems is October 1, 2013. A second rule related to the HIPAA transaction standards—X12 version 5010 and NCPDP (National Council for Prescription Drug Programs) version D.0—establishes earlier effective dates. The HIPAA transactions software must be updated to accommodate the use of the ICD-10-CM and ICD-10-PCS code sets by January 1, 2012, with the exception of Medicaid Pharmacy Subrogation Transactions, which have an effective date of January 1, 2013.

How To Use This Book

Root Operations: Key to Procedure Coding in ICD-10-PCS was primarily designed to focus on the ICD-10-PCS terms and definitions, in addition to presenting current ICD-9-CM cases and procedure codes for comparing and mapping these cases and codes to ICD-10-PCS. *Root Operations: Key to Procedure Coding in ICD-10-PCS* is **not** a text on how to code in ICD-10-PCS nor does it attempt to teach everything there is to transition to ICD-10-PCS. The intent of this book is to provide the coding professional with the groundwork necessary to begin understanding and contrasting procedures coded in ICD-9-CM to those coded in ICD-10-PCS.

It is the coding professional's responsibility to learn ICD-10-PCS terms and definitions and to apply them to correctly assign codes. Learning these definitions is key to identifying the correct ICD-10-PCS code. In the Medical and Surgical section alone, there are 31 Root Operations that must be memorized and understood in order to apply them when coding a procedure.

This text concentrates on the Root Operation (character 3) of ICD-10-PCS because the Root Operation is the critical factor to the correct code assignment. Determining the Root Operation (the intent of the procedure) is the key and illustrates the precision of the code values defined in the ICD-10-PCS system. Chapters 4 through 12 include case excerpts in the section titled "Apply Knowledge to Transition from Coding in ICD-9-CM to ICD-10-PCS."

Furthermore, it is the coding professional's responsibility—not the physician's—to review the clinical documentation in the medical record and equate it to the correct ICD-10-PCS Root Operation. The linking or mapping of ICD-10-PCS definitions to clinical documentation is the coder's responsibility. The physician is not required or expected to use actual terms in ICD-10-PCS code descriptions, nor is the coder required to query the physician when the correlation between the documentation and the defined ICD-10-PCS terms are not provided. For example, when the physician documents removal of a thrombus, the coder would independently correlate "removal of a thrombus" to the Root Operation "Extirpation" using the ICD-10-PCS definitions.

It is not too early for coding professionals to begin learning the various ICD-10-PCS definitions such as the Root Operations and approaches. Progressive learning of ICD-10-PCS will result in a better understanding of ICD-10-PCS when the classification system is implemented. The *Root Operations: Key to Procedure Coding in ICD-10-PCS* is an excellent preparatory text for new or proficient coders, in addition to anyone who needs a solid foundation enabling a steady transition to ICD-10-PCS.

The codes utilized in this book are:

- ICD-9-CM codes and guidelines: 2010 version
- ICD-10-PCS codes: 2010 version
- ICD-10-PCS guidelines: 2011 version

The ICD-10-CM/PCS codes may change for 2012. The 2011 guidelines are available online from CMS: http://www.cms.gov/ICD10/Downloads/PCS2011guidelines.pdf. Please check the CMS Web site for the latest information.

Acknowledgments

The publisher thanks Judy A. Bielby, MBA, RHIA, CPHQ, CCS, for her thoughtful review of Chapter 2.

Portions of this book originally appeared in the following publications:

- Schraffenberger, Lou Ann. 2011. *Basic ICD-9-CM Coding Exercises,* 3rd ed. Chicago: AHIMA.
- AHIMA. 2011. *Clinical Coding Workout.* Chicago: AHIMA.

Chapter 1

Introduction to ICD-10-PCS

The Department of Health and Human Services (HHS) published the final rule adopting ICD-10-CM and ICD-10-PCS as replacements for the ICD-9-CM code set in the January 16, 2009, *Federal Register.* The ICD-10-CM diagnosis codes will be used industry-wide to report diagnosis codes. ICD-10-CM is based on the World Health Organization's (WHO) ICD-10 coding system. Both the WHO version of ICD-10 and the U.S. ICD-10-CM contain diagnostic codes only.

In the United States, the Centers for Medicare & Medicaid Services (CMS) is responsible for maintaining the inpatient procedure code set. CMS contracted with 3M Health Information Systems to design and develop a procedure classification system to replace Volume 3 of ICD-9-CM. ICD-10-PCS was released in 1998, and it will be implemented as the procedural coding system for hospital inpatients October 1, 2013.

Background of ICD-10-PCS

ICD-10-PCS is totally different from ICD-9-CM in structure, organization, and capabilities. During its development, structural attributes were recommended as desirable in a new system. These attributes are:

- Multiaxial structure
- Completeness
- Expandability

Multiaxial Structure

The multiaxial structure of ICD-10-PCS makes it possible for the ICD-10-PCS to be complete, expandable, and to provide a high degree of

1

flexibility and functionality. Each ICD-10-PCS code contains seven characters, with each of those characters representing a category of information specific about the procedure performed. Each position can be thought of as an independent axis. Values are inserted into that stable position in the code and provide specific information about the procedure. This will be discussed later in this chapter.

It is possible to add to values for a character as needed, making ICD-10-PCS expandable and flexible. If new devices or approaches are used, new values can be added to the system.

Completeness

ICD-10-PCS has these exclusive qualities:

- A unique code is available for each significantly different procedure.
- Each code retains its unique definition. Codes are not reused.

In Volume 3 of ICD-9-CM, one assigned procedure code may contain procedures performed on many different body parts using different approaches or devices. In ICD-10-PCS, a unique code can be assigned for every significantly different procedure.

Within each section, a character defines a consistent component of a code that contains all applicable values for that character. Specific values are used for possible values (for example, open, percutaneous). Using the applicable value, unique codes can be constructed. Each character has its unique code because the codes are constructed with individual values rather than from code lists. This quality allows for expandability and retention of the codes. New values can be added, but codes are not given new meanings and reused.

Expandability

Expandability was also considered key to the structure of ICD-10-PCS. A system capable of being easily expanded must accommodate new procedures and technologies and add new codes without disrupting the existing structure.

Changes to ICD-10-PCS can be made within the existing structure because whole codes are not added. ICD-10-PCS provides two unique ways to add changes:

- A new value for a character is added
- An existing value for a character is added to a table(s) in the system

Other Characteristics of ICD-10-PCS

ICD-10-PCS contains other desirable characteristics such as:

- Standardized terminology within the coding system (with no diagnostic information)
- Standardized level of specificity
- No explicit "not otherwise specified" (NOS) code options
- Limited use of "not elsewhere classified" (NEC) code options

Standardized Terminology

Confusion and inaccurate code assignment can result if terms are not well defined. ICD-10-PCS is standardized with characters and values used in the system defined.

The word "Excision" may be used to describe a wide variety of surgical procedures. In ICD-10-PCS, the word "Excision" describes a single, precise surgical objective, defined as "Cutting out or off, without replacement, a portion of a body part."

Because the terminology used in ICD-10-PCS is standardized, no procedure names, diagnostic information, or eponyms are used.

One example is ICD-9-CM code 27.42, "Wide excision of lesion of lip." This procedure includes diagnostic information that a lesion is excised. In code 22.61, "Excision of lesion of maxillary sinus with Caldwell-Luc approach," diagnostic information, and the eponym are included. ICD-9-CM also includes many eponyms in the Index (for example, Collis-Nissen, Davis, Fowler, Kehr, McDonald, and others). Physicians' names are not used in ICD-10-PCS Index or code description. Further procedures are not identified by common terms or acronyms such as cholecystectomy or CABG. Instead, each procedure is coded to the root operation that accurately identifies the objective of the procedure.

In addition, ICD-10-PCS does not typically define multiple procedures with one code. This is to preserve standardized terminology and consistency across the system. A procedure that meets the reporting criteria for a separate procedure (per Coding Guidelines) is coded separately in ICD-10-PCS. This allows the system to respond to changes in technology and medical practice with the maximum degree of stability and flexibility.

Standardized Level of Specificity

ICD-10-PCS provides specificity in the code by representing a single procedure code per procedure. This is vastly different in ICD-9-CM where one code with its description may encompass many procedure variations.

The ICD-9-CM code 39.31, "Suture of artery," does not specify the artery, while in ICD-10-PCS the specific body part is identified by utilizing different codes.

In general, ICD-10-PCS code descriptions are much more specific than their ICD-9-CM counterparts, but sometimes an ICD-10-PCS code description is actually *less* specific. In most cases this is because the ICD-9-CM code contains diagnosis information. Adding diagnostic information limits the flexibility and functionality of a procedure coding system. It has the effect of placing a code "off limits" because the diagnosis in the medical record does not match the diagnosis in the procedure code description. The code cannot be used even though the procedural part of the code description precisely matches the procedure performed. The diagnosis codes, not the procedure codes, will specify the reason the procedure is performed.

NOS and NEC Code Options

ICD-9-CM often designates codes as "unspecified" or "not otherwise specified" codes. In ICD-10-PCS, each character defines information about the procedure and all seven characters must contain a specific value obtained from a single row of a table to build a valid code. When characters such as "Device" and "Qualifier" are not applicable in a code, the character Z is used as the value. Even utilizing this value provides information about the procedure.

ICD-9-CM also designates codes as "not elsewhere classified" or "not other specified" versions of a procedure throughout the code set. NEC options are also provided in ICD-10-PCS, but only for specific, limited use. The root operation value Q, Repair, and the device value Y, Other device, are the NEC values in ICD-10-PCS. These will be discussed later in the book.

Because of many of these new features, ICD-10-PCS code structure results in qualities that optimize the performance of the system in electronic applications, and maximize the usefulness of the coded healthcare data. For example there is optimal search capability in ICD-10-PCS because of the standard meanings and consistent character definitions for each character. These consistent values enable code readability.

Format/Structure of ICD-10-PCS

While ICD-9-CM is a numeric structure of three to four characters, ICD-10-PCS has an entirely new structure. Each code is seven characters, and any character can be alphabetical or numeric. The ten digits 0-9 and the 24 letters A-H, J-N, and P-Z are used. The letters I and O are not used in order to not be confused with the digits 1 and 0. The alpha characters are not case-sensitive. There are no decimal points in ICD-10-PCS.

Each of the seven characters has a well-defined meaning. The characters and meanings change depending on the section in ICD-10-PCS. Figure 1.1 identifies the characters in the Medical/Surgical Section.

Table 1.1 briefly compares ICD-9-CM procedure codes to ICD-10-PCS.

Figure 1.1.   Format and structure of ICD-10-PCS

1	2	3	4	5	6	7
Section	Body System	Root Operation	Body Part	Approach	Device	Qualifier

Table 1.1.   Comparison of ICD-9-CM procedure codes to ICD-10-PCS

ICD-9-CM	ICD-10-PCS
Follows ICD structure	Designed/developed to meet healthcare needs for procedure code system
Codes available as fixed/finite set in list form	Codes constructed from flexible code components (values) using tables
ICD-9-CM has 3–4 characters	ICD-10-PCS has 7 characters
All characters are numeric	Each can be either alpha or numeric
All codes have at least 3 characters	Each code must have 7 characters
Decimal used after second number	No decimals used in system
	Alpha characters are *not* case-sensitive
	Numbers 0–9; letters A–H, J–N, P–Z

Definitions of the 7 Characters in Medical and Surgical Section

Character 1: Section

The first character indicates the section, or the broad procedure category. The sections of ICD-10-PCS are shown in table 1.2.

Table 1.2.   The sections of ICD-10-PCS

Section Value	Description
0	Medical and Surgical
1	Obstetrics
2	Placement
3	Administration
4	Measurement and Monitoring
5	Extracorporeal Assistance and Performance
6	Extracorporeal Therapies
7	Osteopathic
8	Other Procedures
9	Chiropractic
B	Imaging
C	Nuclear Medicine
D	Radiation Oncology
F	Physical Rehabilitation and Diagnostic Audiology
G	Mental Health
H	Substance Abuse Treatment

Character 2: Body System

The second character defines the body part, or the general physiological system or anatomical region involved. This way of categorizing into larger groupings first makes the tables easier to navigate and also provides information quickly about the procedure. All procedures with the same second character would be of the same anatomical region or body part as shown in table 1.3.

Body System Guidelines

B2.1a: The procedure codes in the general anatomical regions body parts should only be used when the procedure is performed on an anatomical region rather than a specific body part (for example, root operations Control and Detachment, drainage of a body cavity) or on the rare occasion when no information is available to support assignment of a code to a specific body part.

> **Example:**   Control of postoperative hemorrhage is coded to the root operation control found in the general anatomical regions body parts.

B2.1b: Body systems designated as Upper or Lower contain body parts located above or below the diaphragm, respectively.

> **Example:**   Vein body parts above the diaphragm are found in the Upper Veins body part; vein body parts below the diaphragm are found in the Lower Veins body part.

Character 3: Root Operation

The third character defines the root operation, or the objective of the procedure. There are 31 root operations in the Medical and Surgical Section, and they are arranged by groups with similar attributes. If multiple procedures as defined by distinct objectives are performed, then multiple codes are assigned.

Examples of root operations are as follows. The complete list is shown in figure 1.2.

- Bypass
- Removal
- Transfer
- Resection
- Destruction

Table 1.3.   Medical and Surgical Section Body Systems

Body System	Value	Body System	Value
Central Nervous	0	Subcutaneous Tissue and Fascia	J
Peripheral Nervous	1	Muscles	K
Heart and Great Vessels	2	Tendons—Includes synovial membrane	L
Upper Arteries	3	Bursae and Ligaments—Includes synovial membrane	M
Lower Arteries	4	Head and Facial Bones	N
Upper Veins	5	Upper Bones	P
Lower Veins	6	Lower Bones	Q
Lymphatic and Hemic—Includes lymph vessels and lymph nodes	7	Upper Joints—Includes synovial membrane	R
Eye	8	Lower Joints—Includes synovial membrane	S
Ear, Nose, Sinus—Includes sinus ducts	9	Urinary	T
Respiratory	B	Female Reproductive	U
Mouth and Throat	C	Male Reproductive	V
Gastrointestinal	D	Anatomical Regions, General	W
Hepatobiliary and Pancreas	F	Anatomical Regions, Upper Extremities	X
Endocrine	G	Anatomical Regions, Lower Extremities	Y
Skin and Breast—Includes skin and breast glands and ducts	H		

Figure 1.2. Medical and Surgical Section Root Operations

Alteration	Division	Inspection	Reposition
Bypass	Drainage	Map	Resection
Change	Excision	Occlusion	Restriction
Control	Extirpation	Reattachment	Revision
Creation	Extraction	Release	Supplement
Destruction	Fragmentation	Removal	Transfer
Detachment	Fusion	Repair	Transplantation
Dilation	Insertion	Replacement	

The general guidelines for root operations are presented later in this chapter, while the root specific guidelines will be presented in the applicable root operation groupings.

Character 4: Body Part

The fourth character defines the body part or specific anatomical site where the procedure was performed. This is the specific site, different from character 2 that provided the general body system. There are 34 possible body part values in each body part.

Examples of body parts are:

- Liver
- Kidney
- Axillary vein, left
- Ascending Colon
- Radial nerve
- Tonsil
- Cerebellum
- Upper lung lobe, right

Body Part Guidelines

General Guidelines

B4.1a: If a procedure is performed on a portion of a body part that does not have a separate body part value, code the body part value corresponding to the whole body part.

> **Example:** A procedure performed on the alveolar process of the mandible is coded to the mandible body part.

B4.1b: If the prefix "peri-" is combined with a body part to identify the site of the procedure, the procedure is coded to the body part named.

> **Example:**   A procedure site identified as perirenal is coded to the kidney body part.

Branches of Body Parts

B4.2: Where a specific branch of a body part does not have its own body part value in PCS, the body part is coded to the closest proximal branch that has a specific body part value.

> **Example:**   A procedure performed on the mandibular branch of the trigeminal nerve is coded to the trigeminal nerve body part value.

Bilateral Body Part Values

B4.3: Bilateral body part values are available for a limited number of body parts. If the identical procedure is performed on contralateral body parts, and a bilateral body part value exists for that body part, a single procedure is coded using the bilateral body part value. If no bilateral body part value exists, each procedure is coded separately using the appropriate body part value.

> **Example:**   The identical procedure performed on both fallopian tubes is coded once using the body part value Fallopian Tube, Bilateral. The identical procedure performed on both knee joints is coded twice using the body part values Knee Joint, Right and Knee Joint, Left.

Coronary Arteries

B4.4: The coronary arteries are classified as a single body part that is further specified by number of sites treated and not by name or number of arteries. Separate body part values are used to specify the number of sites treated when the same procedure is performed on multiple sites in the coronary arteries.

> **Examples:**   1. Angioplasty of two distinct sites in the left anterior descending coronary artery with placement of two stents is coded as Dilation of Coronary Arteries, Two Sites, with Intraluminal Device.

2. Angioplasty of two distinct sites in the left anterior descending coronary artery, one with stent placed and one without, is coded separately as Dilation of Coronary Artery, One Site with Intraluminal Device, and Dilation of Coronary Artery, One Site with no Device.

Tendons, Ligaments, Bursae, and Fascia near a Joint

B4.5: Procedures performed on tendons, ligaments, bursae, and fascia supporting a joint are coded to the body part in the respective body system that is the focus of the procedure. Procedures performed on joint structures themselves are coded to the body part in the joint body parts.

Example: Repair of the anterior cruciate ligament of the knee is coded to the knee bursae and ligament body part in the bursae and ligaments body system. Knee arthroscopy with shaving of articular cartilage is coded to the knee joint body part in the Lower Joints body part.

Skin, Subcutaneous Tissue, and Fascia Overlying a Joint

B4.6: If a procedure is performed on the skin, subcutaneous tissue, or fascia overlying a joint, the procedure is coded to the following body part:

- Shoulder is coded to Upper Arm
- Elbow is coded to Lower Arm
- Wrist is coded to Lower Arm
- Hip is coded to Upper Leg
- Knee is coded to Lower Leg
- Ankle is coded to Foot

Fingers and Toes

B4.7: If a body part does not contain a separate body part value for fingers, procedures performed on the fingers are coded to the body part value for the hand. If a body part does not contain a separate body part value for toes, procedures performed on the toes are coded to the body part value for the foot.

Example: Excision of finger muscle is coded to one of the hand muscle body part values in the Muscles body part.

Character 5: Approach

The fifth character defines the Approach: the technique used to reach the procedure site. There are seven different Approach values in the Medical and Surgical section. The approach character is discussed in more detail in Chapter 3.

Character 6: Device

There may or may not be a Device left in place, depending on the procedure performed. The sixth character identifies these Devices. Device values fall into four basic groups:

- Grafts and Prostheses
- Implants
- Simple or Mechanical Appliances
- Electronic Appliances

Note: Devices
Only procedures in which a device remains after the procedure is completed will have a specific Device value assigned. Remember that all codes require seven characters. The default value to indicate that **NO** device was involved is **Z**.

Examples of Device values:

- Drainage device
- Radioactive element
- Autologous tissue substitute
- Extraluminal device
- Intraluminal device
- Synthetic substitute
- Nonautologous tissue substitute

Note: Materials incidental to a procedure such as clips, sutures, ligatures, radiological markers, and temporary post-operative wound drains are considered integral to the performance of the procedure and are not coded as devices.

Device Guidelines

General Guidelines

B6.1a: A Device is coded only if a Device remains after the procedure is completed. If no Device remains, the Device value No Device is coded.

B6.1b: Materials such as sutures, ligatures, radiological markers, and temporary post-operative wound drains are considered integral to the performance of a procedure and are not coded as Devices.

B6.1c: Procedures performed on a Device only and not on a Body Part are specified in the Root Operations Change, Irrigation, Removal, and Revision, and are coded to the procedure performed.

> **Example:**   Irrigation of percutaneous nephrostomy tube is coded to the root operation Irrigation of indwelling device in the Administration section.

Drainage Device

B6.2: A separate procedure to put in a drainage device is coded to the Root Operation Drainage with the device value Drainage Device.

Character 7: Qualifier

The seventh character defines a Qualifier for the code that provides additional information about a specific attribute of the procedure. These Qualifiers may have a narrow application, such as to a specific root operation, body system, or body part.

Examples of Qualifiers

- Type of transplant
- Second site for a bypass
- Diagnostic excision (biopsy)

Note: Qualifier
Most procedures will not have an applicable qualifier. The default value to indicate that **NO** qualifier is needed is **Z**.

Guidelines

The ICD-10-PCS Draft Coding Guidelines (2011) are available for review. There are three main sections of Guidelines:

A.   Conventions
B.   Medical and Surgical Section Guidelines (section 0)
C.   Obstetrics Section Guidelines

Section B is by far the most extensive section. There are guidelines for:

• Body System
• Root Operation
• Body Part
• Approach
• Device

An effort has been made to incorporate the Medical and Surgical Section Approach and Root Operation Guidelines into the applicable areas in this book, but the General Guidelines have overarching principals that must be understood before proceeding. Specific Medical and Surgical Section Guidelines for body system, body part, and Device were discussed previously in this chapter.

Conventions

A1: ICD-10-PCS codes are composed of seven characters. Each character is an axis of classification that specifies information about the procedure performed. Within a defined code range, a character specifies the same type of information in that axis of classification.

> **Example:** The fifth axis of classification specifies the approach in sections 0 through 4 and 7 through 9 of the system.

A2: One of 34 possible values can be assigned to each axis of classification in the seven-character code: they are the numbers 0 through 9 and the alphabet (except I and O because they are easily confused with the numbers 1 and 0). The number of unique values used in an axis of classification differs as needed.

> **Example:** Where the fifth axis of classification specifies the approach, seven different approach values are currently used to specify the approach.

A3: The valid values for an axis of classification can be added to as needed.

> **Example:**   If a significantly distinct type of device is used in a new procedure, a new device value can be added to the system.

A4: As with words in their context, the meaning of any single value is a combination of its axis of classification and any preceding values on which it may be dependent.

> **Example:**   The meaning of a body part value in the Medical and Surgical section is always dependent on the body system value. The body part value 0 in the Central Nervous body system specifies Brain, and the body part value 0 in the Peripheral Nervous body system specifies Cervical Plexus.

A5: As the system is expanded as needed to include increasing detail, the values will depend on preceding values for their meaning.

> **Example:**   In the Lower Joints body system, the Device value 3 in the Root Operation Insertion specifies Infusion Device, and the Device value 3 in the Root Operation Fusion specifies Interbody Fusion Device.

A6: The purpose of the alphabetic index is to locate the appropriate table that contains all information necessary to construct a procedure code. The PCS tables should always be consulted to find the most appropriate valid code.

A7: It is not required to consult the Index before proceeding to the tables to complete the code. A valid code may be chosen directly from the tables.

A8: All seven characters must be specified to be a valid code. If the documentation is incomplete for coding purposes, the physician should be queried for the necessary information.

A9: Within a PCS Table, valid codes include all combinations of choices in characters 4 through 7 contained in the same row of the Table. As shown in figure 1.3, 0JHT3VZ is a valid code, and 0JHW3VZ is *not* a valid code.

Figure 1.3.   Example of a valid code and an invalid code

0JHT3VZ is a valid code. 0JHW3VZ is *not* a valid code

Section:	0	Medical and Surgical
Body System:	**J**	Subcutaneous Tissue and Fascia
Operation:	**H**	Insertion: Putting in a nonbiological appliance that monitors, assists, performs, or prevents a physiological function but does not physically take the place of a body part

Body Part	Approach	Device	Qualifier
S Subcutaneous Tissue and Fascia, Head and Neck **V** Subcutaneous Tissue and Fascia, Upper Extremity **W** Subcutaneous Tissue and Fascia, Lower Extremity	**0** Open **3** Percutaneous	**1** Radioactive Element **3** Infusion Device	**Z** No Qualifier
T Subcutaneous Tissue and Fascia, Trunk	**0** Open **3** Percutaneous	**1** Radioactive Element **3** Infusion Device **V** Infusion Pump	**Z** No Qualifier

A10: "And," when used in a code description, means "and/or."

> **Example:** Lower Arm and Wrist Muscle means lower arm and/or wrist muscle.

A11: Many of the terms used to construct PCS codes are defined within the system. It is the coder's responsibility to determine what the documentation in the medical record equates to in the PCS definitions. The physician is not expected to use the terms used in PCS code descriptions, nor is the coder required to query the physician when the correlation between the documentation and the defined PCS terms is clear.

> **Example:** When the physician documents "partial resection" the coder can independently correlate "partial resection" to the root operation Excision without querying the physician for clarification.

Alphabetical Index and Tables

The structure of the Index and Tabular List is very different from ICD-9-CM procedure coding. The Index provides a limited number of characters, so it is necessary to go to the Table to find all characters. Sometimes, however, all seven characters are provided in the Index.

Index

The ICD-10-PCS Index can be used to access the Tables. The Index is organized as an alphabetic lookup, which provides at least the first three characters of the code (sometimes more). After obtaining this information, the Table is consulted to select the rest of the characters. It is possible to construct a code by going directly to a Table, and this is permitted.

Main index term is a Root Operation, root procedure type, or common procedure name. Examples are:

- Bypass (Root Operation)
- Fluoroscopy (root type)
- Appendectomy (common procedure name)

Tables

The Tables are a grid with rows and columns to select valid combinations of code characters. The Tables are organized in a series, beginning with section 0 (Medical/Surgical) and Body System 0 (Central Nervous), and proceeding in numerical order. Sections 0 through 9 are then followed by sections B through D and F through H. This same organization is followed within each table for the second through seventh characters— numeric values in order, followed by alphabetical values in order.

The Medical and Surgical section is organized by the 31 Body System values. The values for characters 1 through 3 are provided at the top of the table. Four columns contain the applicable values for characters 4 through 7, given the values in characters 1 through 3.

The Table may be separated into rows to specify the valid choices of values in characters 4 through 7. A code built using values from more than one row of a table is NOT a valid code. When reviewing the Tables, sometimes there are multiple Tables for the first three characters, and they may cover multiple pages (either on the computer screen or in a code book).

Figures 1.4 and 1.5 provide examples of the Index and Tables.

Figure 1.4.   Open resection of descending colon (complete)

Step 1
Look up term in Alphabetic Index:
Resection
  Colon
    Ascending 0DTK
    Descending 0DTM
    Sigmoid 0DTN
    Transverse 0DTL

Step 2
Proceed to the Table (0DTM)

Section	0	Medical and Surgical
Body System	**D**	Gastrointestinal System
Operation	**T**	Resection: Cutting out or off, without replacement, all of a body part

Body Part	Approach	Device	Qualifier
1 Esophagus, Upper 2 Esophagus, Middle 3 Esophagus, Lower 4 Esophagogastric Junction 5 Esophagus 6 Stomach 7 Stomach, Pylorus 8 Small Intestine 9 Duodenum A Jejunum B Ileum C Ileocecal Valve E Large Intestine F Large Intestine, Right G Large Intestine, Left H Cecum J Appendix K Ascending Colon L Transverse Colon M Descending Colon N Sigmoid Colon P Rectum Q Anus	0 Open 4 Percutaneous Endoscopic 7 Via Natural or Artificial Opening 8 Via Natural or Artificial Opening Endoscopic	Z No Device	Z No Qualifier
R Anal Sphincter S Greater Omentum T Lesser Omentum	0 Open 4 Percutaneous Endoscopic	Z No Device	Z No Qualifier

CODE: 0DTM0ZZ

In figure 1.4, Table 0DT indicates that the procedure is Medical and Surgical, that the Body System is Gastrointestinal, and that the Root Operation is Resection. Resection is defined as Cutting out or off, without replacement, all of a body part.

The fourth character M, indicates that the Body Part is Descending Colon. Because this value is found in the top ROW of the Table, it is necessary to continue coding across the columns in this row. It is incorrect to select any values from the bottom row. The complete code assignment is listed below.

1. Section—Medical and Surgical—0
2. Body system—Gastrointestinal System—D
3. Root Operation—Resection—T
4. Body Part—Descending Colon—M
5. Approach—Open—0
6. Device—No Device—Z
7. Qualifier—No Qualifier—Z

0DTM0ZZ

In figure 1.5, Table 0HB indicates that the procedure is Medical and Surgical, that the Body System is Skin and Breast, and that the Root Operation is Excision. Excision is defined as Cutting out or off, without replacement, a portion of a body part.

The fourth character U indicates that the Body Part is Breast, Left. Because this value is found in the bottom ROW of the Table, it is necessary to continue coding across in this row. It is incorrect to select values from the top row. The complete code assignment is listed below.

1. Section—Medical and Surgical—0
2. Body system—Skin and Breast—H
3. Root Operation—Excision—B
4. Body Part—Breast, Left—U
5. Approach—Percutaneous—3
6. Device—No Device—Z
7. Qualifier—Diagnostic—X (in ICD-10-PCS a biopsy is coded diagnostic—X)

0HBU3ZX

Figure 1.5.   Needle biopsy left breast mass

Step 1

Look up term in Alphabetic Index:
Biopsy
See Drainage, Diagnostic
***See* Excision, Diagnostic**
In this case Excision is selected because there is no documentation that a drainage was done but rather that there was a biopsy done of a mass.
Excision
   Breast
      Bilateral 0HBV
      Left 0HBU
      Right 0HBT
      Supernumerary 0HBY

Step 2

Proceed to the Table

Section	**0**	Medical and Surgical
Body System	**H**	Skin and Breast
Operation	**B**	Excision: Cutting out or off, without replacement, a portion of a body part

Body Part	Approach	Device	Qualifier
0 Skin, Scalp **1** Skin, Face **2** Skin, Right Ear **3** Skin, Left Ear **4** Skin, Neck **5** Skin, Chest **6** Skin, Back **7** Skin, Abdomen **8** Skin, Buttock **9** Skin, Perineum **A** Skin, Genitalia **B** Skin, Right Upper Arm **C** Skin, Left Upper Arm **D** Skin, Right Lower Arm **E** Skin, Left Lower Arm **F** Skin, Right Hand **G** Skin, Left Hand **H** Skin, Right Upper Leg **J** Skin, Left Lower Leg **K** Skin, Right Lower Leg **L** Skin, Left Lower Leg **M** Skin, Right Foot **N** Skin, Left Foot **Q** Finger Nail **R** Toe Nail	**X** External	**Z** No Device	**X** Diagnostic **Z** No Qualifier
T Breast, Right **U** Breast, Left **V** Breast, Bilateral **W** Nipple, Right **X** Nipple, Left **Y** Supernumerary Breast	**0** Open **3** Percutaneous **7** Via Natural or Artificial Opening **8** Via Natural or Artificial Opening Endoscopic **X** External	**Z** No Device	**X** Diagnostic **Z** No Qualifier

CODE: 0HBU3ZX

Importance of Clinical Documentation in Coding with ICD-10-PCS

Careful review of the operative report is critical in coding in ICD-10-PCS. Each code requires each of the seven characters to be assigned. When reviewing the two previous examples, it is evident that some values are easy to determine. Determining the Body Part, for instance, is a matter of selecting the specific Body Part in ICD-10-PCS that is the closest site. For the example of the breast biopsy, the left breast was selected as the Body Part. When ICD-10-PCS does not list all Body Parts, guidelines direct the assignment of the character value. For example, when coding nerves and vessels (veins and arteries) a limited number of Body Part values are available. Nerves and vessels that are not identified by a separate Body Part value are coded to the closest proximal branch identified by a body part values.

> **Example:** A procedure performed on the mandibular branch of the trigeminal nerve is coded to the Trigeminal Nerve body part value.

When assigning the Root Operation (character 3), it is necessary to determine the intent of the procedure(s). This book focuses on learning the Root Operations in order to apply them correctly.

The Approach values are also included in each coded procedure, so identifying the approach from the clinical documentation is required.

Further, in order to interpret Root Operations, Devices, and Qualifiers, it is important that the coding professional utilize knowledge of anatomy and physiology, and knowledge about how the surgical procedure was performed.

Terminology Changes in ICD-10-PCS

Because ICD-10-PCS terms are well defined, it is the coder's responsibility to learn these terms and apply them to correctly assign codes. Learning the definitions is key to coding correctly in this system. In the Medical and Surgical section alone, there are 31 Root Operations that must be memorized and understood in order to apply them to coding a procedure. This book focuses on those definitions and presents examples of current ICD-9-CM cases/codes in order to prepare the coding professional for the transition to ICD-10-PCS. This book does not attempt to teach everything there is to know about ICD-10-PCS nor to attempt to code ICD-10-PCS cases. That is the next step. The intent of this book is to provide the groundwork necessary to take that next step.

The ICD-10-PCS Draft Coding Guidelines and the actual coding system (including the Index and Tables) are readily available at the CMS Web site (www.cms.gov/ICD10). While not necessary to proceed through this text, one might consider it helpful to access the coding system and guidelines before attempting to assign ICD-10-PCS codes.

Further, many terms used to construct ICD-10-PCS codes are defined in the system, and it is the coder's responsibility to determine what the documentation in the medical record equates to in the ICD-10-PCS definitions. The coding professional makes that map or link. The physician is not expected to use the actual terms used in ICD-10-PCS code descriptions, nor is the coder required to query the physician when the correlation between the documentation and the defined ICD-10-PCS terms are not provided. For example, when the physician documents "partial resection," the coder would independently correlate "partial resection" to the Root Operation "Excision" using the ICD-10-PCS definitions.

Physicians use terms interchangeably, and the coding professional must interpret terms such as "removal," "excision," "resection," or "extraction" into the correct ICD-10-PCS root operation based upon the definitions.

Introduction to Root Operations

Root Operation was briefly discussed above. Character 3 in ICD-10-PCS identifies the objective of each procedure. It is really the heart of the entire coding system. Determining the Root Operation is the key and illustrates the precision of the code values defined in the system. There is clear distinction between each Root Operation. In the Medical and Surgical section alone, there are 31 Root Operations. This text will explain each root and provide practice in applying that concept.

Root Operation Guidelines

General Guidelines

B3.1a: In order to determine the appropriate root operation, the full definition of the Root Operation as contained in the PCS Tables must be applied.

B3.1b: Components of a procedure specified in the Root Operation definition and explanation are not coded separately. Procedural steps necessary to reach the operative site and close the operative site are also not coded separately.

> **Example:** Resection of a joint as part of a joint replacement procedure is included in the Root Operation definition of Replacement and is not coded separately. Laparotomy performed to reach the site of an open liver biopsy is not coded separately.

Multiple Procedures

B3.2: During the same operative episode, multiple procedures are coded if:

a. The same root operation is performed on different body parts as defined by distinct values of the body part character.

> **Example:** Diagnostic excision of liver and pancreas are coded separately.

b. The same root operation is repeated at different body sites that are included in the same body part value.

> **Example:** Excision of the sartorius muscle and excision of the gracilis muscle are both included in the upper leg muscle Body Part value, and multiple procedures are coded.

c. Multiple root operations with distinct objectives are performed on the same body part.

> **Example:** Destruction of sigmoid lesion and bypass of sigmoid colon are coded separately.

d. The intended root operation is attempted using one approach, but is converted to a different approach.

> **Example:** Laparoscopic cholecystectomy converted to an open chole-cystectomy is coded as percutaneous endoscopic Inspection and open Resection.

Discontinued Procedures

B3.3: If the intended procedure is discontinued, code the procedure to the root operation performed. If a procedure is discontinued before any other root operation is performed, code the root operation Inspection of the body part or anatomical region inspected.

> **Example:**   A planned aortic valve replacement procedure is discontinued after the initial thoracotomy and before any incision is made in the heart muscle, when the patient becomes hemodynamically unstable. This procedure is coded as an open Inspection of the mediastinum.

Biopsy Followed by more Definitive Treatment

B3.4: If a diagnostic Excision, Extraction, or Drainage procedure (biopsy) is followed by a more definitive procedure—such as Destruction, Excision, or Resection—at the same procedure site, both the biopsy and the more definitive treatment are coded.

> **Example:**   Biopsy of breast is followed by partial mastectomy at the same procedure site. Both the biopsy and the partial mastectomy procedure are coded.

Overlapping Body Layers

B3.5: If the root operations Excision, Repair, or Inspection are performed on overlapping layers of the musculoskeletal system, the body part specifying the deepest layer is coded.

> **Example:**   Excisional debridement that includes skin and subcutaneous tissue and muscle is coded to the muscle body part.

Note: The specific Root Operation Guidelines (B3.6a through B3.16) will be presented in the appropriate section of this text.

The 31 root operations are arranged into the following groupings:

- Root operations that take out some/all of a body part
- Root operations that take out solids/fluids/gases from a body part
- Root operations involving cutting or separation only
- Root operations that put in/put back or move some/all of a body part

- Root operations that alter the diameter/route of a tubular body part
- Root operations that always involve a device
- Root operations involving examination only
- Root operations that include other repairs
- Root operations that include other objectives

These groupings and the specific root operations within these group-ings are discussed in detail in subsequent chapters of this book.

Chapter 2

Snapshot of Anatomy and Physiology for ICD-10-PCS

Central and Peripheral Nervous System

In ICD-10-PCS the body systems available for this system include: Central Nervous System and Peripheral Nervous System. The central nervous system consists of the brain and the spinal cord, while the peripheral nervous system refers to the nerves and ganglia outside the brain and the spinal cord.

In ICD-10-PCS, the structures of the central nervous system affecting procedural code assignment are listed in figure 2.1.

ICD-10-PCS does not list every anatomical site in the body part character values. For this reason, ICD-10-PCS provides a bridge called a body part key. For example, the third ventricle is identified as a part of the brain, but it is not included as a specific body part in ICD-10-PCS. Using the body part key by Anatomical Term, the third ventricle is considered to be in the cerebral ventricle body part. The lobes of the cerebrum (frontal, parietal, temporal, and occipital) are classified to the cerebral hemisphere in ICD-10-PCS. It is advisable that coding professionals reference anatomy resources to increase their knowledge in the preparation for coding in ICD-10-PCS.

Figure 2.1.   Structures of the central nervous system

Brain	Pons	Acoustic nerve
Cerebral meninges	Cerebellum	Glossopharyngeal nerve
Dura mater	Medulla oblongata	Vagus nerve
Epidural space	Cranial nerve	Accessory nerve
Subdural space	Olfactory nerve	Hypoglossal nerve
Subarachnoid space	Optic nerve	Spinal meninges
Cerebral ventricle	Oculomotor nerve	Spinal canal
Cerebral hemisphere	Trochlear nerve	Spinal cord
Basal ganglia	Trigeminal nerve	Cervical spinal cord
Thalamus	Abducens nerve	Thoracic spinal cord
Hypothalamus	Facial nerve	Lumbar spinal cord

For the peripheral nervous system, the body part values available include the following: the cervical plexus, cervical nerve, phrenic nerve, brachial plexus, ulnar nerve, median nerve, radial nerve, thoracic nerve, lumbar plexus, lumbosacral plexus, lumbar nerve, pudendal nerve, femoral nerve, sciatic nerve, tibial nerve, peroneal nerve, head and neck sympathetic nerve, thoracic sympathetic nerve, abdominal sympathetic nerve, lumbar sympathetic nerve, sacral sympathetic nerve, sacral plexus, sacral nerve, and peripheral nerve.

The peripheral nervous system is divided into the autonomic and somatic nervous system. The autonomic division includes the enteric, parasympathetic, and sympathetic subdivisions and the somatic division includes the cranial and spinal nerves and their ganglia and the peripheral sensory receptors.

ICD-10-PCS Body Part Key

The ICD-10-PCS terms used to describe a body part may correspond to anatomical terms. To bridge the two, consult tables 2.1 and 2.2.

Table 2.1.   Central Nervous System Body Part key by ICD-10-PCS description

ICD-10-PCS Term	Anatomical Term(s)
Abducens nerve	Sixth cranial nerve
Accessory nerve	Eleventh cranial nerve
Acoustic nerve	Cochlear nerve, Eighth cranial nerve, Scarpa's (vestibular) ganglion, Spiral ganglion, Vestibular (Scarpa's) ganglion, Vestibular nerve, Vestibulocochlear nerve
Basal ganglia	Basal nuclei, Claustrum, Corpus striatum, Globus pallidus, Substantia nigra, Subthalamic nucleus
Brain	Cerebrum, Corpus callosum, Encephalon
Cerebellum	Culmen
Cerebral hemisphere	Frontal lobe, Occipital lobe, Parietal lobe, Temporal lobe
Cerebral meninges	Arachnoid mater, Leptomeninges, Pia mater
Cerebral ventricle	Aqueduct of Sylvius, Cerebral aqueduct (Sylvius), Choroid plexus, Ependyma, Foramen of Monro (intraventricular), Fourth ventricle, Interventricular foramen (Monro), Left lateral ventricle, Right lateral ventricle, Third ventricle

Table 2.1.   (Continued)

ICD-10-PCS Term	Anatomical Term(s)
Dura mater	Cranial dura mater, Dentate ligament, Diaphragma sellae, Falx cerebri, Spinal dura mater, Tentorium cerebelli
Epidural space	Cranial epidural space, Extradural space, Spinal epidural space
Facial nerve	Chorda tympani, Geniculate ganglion, Greater superficial petrosal nerve, Nerve to the stapedius, Parotid plexus, Posterior auricular nerve, Seventh cranial nerve, Submandibular ganglion
Glossopharyngeal nerve	Carotid sinus nerve, Ninth cranial nerve, Tympanic nerve
Hypoglossal nerve	Twelfth cranial nerve
Hypothalamus	Mammillary body
Lumbar spinal cord	Cauda equine, Conus medullaris
Medulla oblongata	Myelencephalon
Oculomotor nerve	Third cranial nerve
Olfactory nerve	First cranial nerve, Olfactory bulb
Optic nerve	Optic chiasma, Second cranial nerve
Pons	Apneustic center, Basis pontis, Locus ceruleus, Pneumotaxic center, Pontine tegmentum, Superior olivary nucleus
Spinal canal	Vertebral canal
Spinal cord	Denticulate ligament
Spinal meninges	Arachnoid mater, Leptomeninges, Pia mater
Subarachnoid space	Cranial subarachnoid space, Spinal subarachnoid space
Subdural space	Cranial subdural space, Spinal subdural space
Thalamus	Epithalamus, Geniculate nucleus, Metathalamus, Pulvinar
Trigeminal nerve	Fifth cranial nerve, Gasserian ganglion, Mandibular nerve, Maxillary nerve, Ophthalmic nerve, Trifacial nerve
Trochlear nerve	Fourth cranial nerve
Vagus nerve	Anterior vagal trunk, Pharyngeal plexus, Pneumogastric nerve, Posterior vagal trunk, Pulmonary plexus, Recurrent laryngeal nerve, Superior laryngeal nerve, Tenth cranial nerve

Table 2.2.   Peripheral Nervous System Body Part key by ICD-10-PCS description

ICD-10-PCS Term	Anatomical Term(s)
Abdominal sympathetic nerve	Abdominal aortic plexus, Auerbach's (myenteric) plexus, Celiac (solar) plexus, Celiac ganglion, Gastric plexus, Hepatic plexus, Inferior hypogastric plexus, Inferior mesenteric plexus, Inferior mesenteric ganglion, Meissner's (submucous) plexus, Myenteric (Auerbach's) plexus, Pancreatic plexus, Pelvic splanchnic nerve, Renal plexus, Solar (celiac) plexus, Splenic plexus, Submucous (Meissner's) plexus, Superior hypogastric plexus, Superior mesenteric plexus, Superior mesenteric ganglion, Suprarenal plexus
Brachial plexus	Axillary nerve, Dorsal scapular nerve, First intercostal nerve, Long thoracic nerve, Musculocutaneous nerve, Subclavius nerve, Suprascapular nerve
Cervical nerve	Greater occipital nerve, Suboccipital nerve, Third occipital nerve
Cervical plexus	Ansa cervicalis, Cutaneous (transverse) cervical nerve, Great auricular nerve, Lesser occipital nerve, Supra-clavicular nerve, Transverse (cutaneous) cervical nerve
Femoral nerve	Anterior crural nerve, Saphenous nerve
Head and neck sympathetic nerve	Cavernous plexus, Cervical ganglion, Ciliary ganglion, Internal carotid plexus, Otic ganglion, Pterygopalatine (sphenopalatine) ganglion, Sphenopalatine (pterygopalatine) ganglion, Stellate ganglion, Submandibular ganglion, Submaxillary ganglion
Lumbar nerve	Lumbosacral trunk, Superior clunic (cluneal) nerve
Lumbar plexus	Accessory obturator nerve, Genitofemoral nerve, Iliohypogastric nerve, Ilioinguinal nerve, Lateral femoral cutaneous nerve, Obturator nerve, Superior gluteal nerve
Lumbar sympathetic nerve	Lumbar ganglion, Lumbar splanchnic nerve
Median nerve	Anterior interosseous nerve, Palmar cutaneous nerve

Table 2.2.   (Continued)

ICD-10-PCS Term	Anatomical Term(s)
Peroneal nerve	Common fibular nerve, Common peroneal nerve, External popliteal nerve, Lateral sural cutaneous nerve
Phrenic nerve	Accessory phrenic nerve
Pudendal nerve	Posterior labial nerve, Posterior scrotal nerve
Radial nerve	Dorsal digital nerve, Musculospiral nerve, Palmar cutaneous nerve, Posterior interosseous nerve
Sacral plexus	Inferior gluteal nerve, Posterior femoral cutaneous nerve, Pudendal nerve
Sacral sympathetic nerve	Ganglion impar (ganglion of Walther), Pelvic splanchnic nerve, Sacral ganglion, Sacral splanchnic nerve
Sciatic nerve	Ischiatic nerve
Thoracic nerve	Intercostal nerve, Intercostobrachial nerve, Subcostal nerve
Thoracic sympathetic nerve	Cardiac plexus, Esophageal plexus, Greater splanchnic nerve, Inferior cardiac nerve, Least splanchnic nerve, Lesser splanchnic nerve, Middle cardiac nerve, Pulmonary plexus, Superior cardiac nerve, Thoracic aortic plexus, Thoracic ganglion
Tibial nerve	Lateral plantar nerve, Medial plantar nerve, Medial popliteal nerve, Medial sural cutaneous nerve
Ulnar nerve	Cubital nerve

Circulatory System

In ICD-10-PCS the body systems available for the circulatory system include: heart and great vessels, arteries, and veins. The heart consists of cardiac muscle that serves as a pump to maintain the circulation of the blood, while the arteries carry the blood away from the heart and the veins are the vessels carrying blood to the heart.

In ICD-10-PCS, the general structures of the heart and great vessels affecting procedural code assignment include the following: coronary artery, coronary vein, atrial septum, atrium, conduction mechanism, chordae tendineae, heart, papillary muscle, aortic valve, mitral valve, pulmonary valve, tricuspid valve, ventricle, ventricular septum, pericardium, pulmonary trunk, pulmonary artery, pulmonary vein, superior vena cava, thoracic aorta, and great vessel. Several of these values include laterality.

Individual body system values are available for upper arteries, lower arteries, upper veins, and lower veins. For the upper arteries, the body part values available in ICD-10-PCS include the following: internal mammary artery, innominate artery, subclavian artery, axillary artery, brachial artery, ulnar artery, radial artery, hand artery, intracranial artery, common carotid artery, internal carotic artery, external carotic artery, vertebral artery, face artery, temporal artery, thyroid artery, and upper artery. Once again, laterality is available when applicable in upper and lower arteries and upper and lower veins.

For the lower arteries, the body part values available in ICD-10-PCS include the following: abdominal aorta, celiac artery, gastric artery, hepatic artery, splenic artery, superior mesenteric artery, colic artery, renal artery, inferior mesenteric artery, common iliac artery, internal iliac artery, external iliac artery, femoral artery, popliteal artery, anterior tibial artery, posterior tibial artery, peroneal artery, foot artery, and lower artery.

For the upper veins, the body part values available in ICD-10-PCS include the following: azygos vein, hemiazygos vein, innominate vein, subclavian vein, axillary vein, brachial vein, basilic vein, cephalic vein, hand vein, intracranial vein, internal jugular vein, external jugular vein, vertebral vein, face vein, and upper vein.

For the lower veins, the body part values available in ICD-10-PCS include the following: inferior vena cava, splenic vein, gastric vein, esophageal vein, hepatic vein, superior mesenteric vein, inferior mesenteric vein, colic vein, portal vein, renal vein, common iliac vein, external iliac vein, hypogastric vein, femoral vein, greater saphenous vein, lesser saphenous vein, foot vein, and lower vein.

The heart is divided into four cavities, right and left atria and right and left ventricles. The right and left sides of the heart are divided by the septum. The atria are divided by the atrial or interatrial septum, and the ventricles are divided by the ventricular or interventricular septum. Blood enters the right atrium from the superior and inferior vena cavae. Blood is pumped into the right ventricle and then pumped to the lungs via pulmonary arteries. In the lungs, oxygen is added to blood and carbon dioxide is passed from the blood. Oxygenated blood comes from the lungs through the pulmonary veins and into the left atrium. The blood then is pumped into the left ventricle, which pumps the blood to the body through the aorta. The heart valves allow the blood to flow in only one direction. The four heart valves are: aortic, tricuspid, pulmonary, and mitral valve.

The cardiac conduction system (also called the electrical system) is made up of three parts:

1. Sinoatrial (SA) node, in the right atrium
2. Atrioventricular (AV) node, in the interatrial septum close to the tricuspid valve
3. His-Purkinje system, located in the walls of the ventricles

The heart and blood vessels make up the blood circulatory system. The arterial circulation consists of the arteries including the aorta and pulmonary arteries. These blood vessels carry blood away from the heart. Healthy arteries should be strong and elastic, becoming narrow between beats of the heart. This keeps blood pressure consistent and helps blood circulate through the body. Smaller branches are arterioles. The venous circulation system carries blood to the heart and includes the vena cavae and pulmonary veins. The veins have thinner walls than arteries and have the ability to widen as blood flow increases. Capillaries then connect the arterial and venous circulation. Capillaries are very small blood vessels and have thin walls, allowing oxygen and nutrients in the blood to pass through the walls into the body. The capillaries likewise absorb carbon dioxide to be transported to the lungs.

ICD-10-PCS Body Part Key

The ICD-10-PCS terms used to describe a body part may correspond to anatomical terms. To bridge the two, consult tables 2.3 through 2.7.

Table 2.3. Heart and Great Vessels Body Part key by ICD-10-PCS description

ICD-10-PCS Term	Anatomical Term(s)
Aortic valve	Aortic annulus
Atrial septum	Interatrial septum
Atrium, left	Atrium pulmonale, Left auricular appendix
Atrium, right	Atrium dextrum cordis, Right auricular appendix, Sinus venosus
Conduction mechanism	Atrioventricular node, Bundle of His, Bundle of Kent, Sinoatrial node
Heart	Interatrial septum
Heart, left	Left coronary sulcus, Obtuse margin
Heart, right	Right coronary sulcus
Mitral valve	Bicuspid valve, Left atrioventricular valve, Mitral annulus
Pulmonary valve	Pulmonary annulus, Pulmonic valve
Pulmonary vein, left	Left inferior pulmonary vein, Left superior pulmonary vein
Pulmonary vein, right	Right inferior pulmonary vein, Right superior pulmonary vein
Superior vena cava	Precava
Thoracic aorta	Aortic arch, Aortic intercostal artery, Ascending aorta, Bronchial artery, Esophageal artery, Subcostal artery
Tricuspid valve	Right atrioventricular valve, Tricuspid annulus
Ventricle, right	Acute margin, Conus arteriosus
Ventricular septum	Interventricular septum

Table 2.4   Upper Arteries Body Part key by ICD-10-PCS description

ICD-10-PCS Term	Anatomical Term(s)
Axillary artery	Anterior circumflex humeral artery, Lateral thoracic artery, Posterior circumflex humeral artery, Subscapular artery, Superior thoracic artery, Thoracoacromial artery
Brachial artery	Inferior ulnar collateral artery, Profunda brachii, Superior ulnar collateral artery
External carotid artery	Ascending pharyngeal artery, Internal maxillary artery, Lingual artery, Maxillary artery, Occipital artery, Posterior auricular artery, Superior thyroid artery
Face artery	Angular artery, Ascending palatine artery, External maxillary artery, Facial artery, Inferior labial artery, Submental artery, Superior labial artery
Hand artery	Deep palmar arch, Princeps pollicis artery, Radialis indicis, Superficial palmar arch
Innominate artery	Brachiocephalic trunk, Brachiocephalic artery
Internal carotid artery	Caroticotympanic artery, Carotid sinus, Ophthalmic artery
Internal mammary artery	Anterior intercostal artery, Internal thoracic artery, Musculophrenic artery, Pericardiophrenic artery, Superior epigastric artery
Intracranial artery	Anterior cerebral artery, Anterior choroidal artery, Anterior communicating artery, Basilar artery, Circle of Willis, Middle cerebral artery, Posterior cerebral artery, Posterior communicating artery, Posterior inferior cerebellar artery (PICA)
Radial artery	Radial recurrent artery
Subclavian artery	Costocervical trunk, Dorsal scapular artery, Internal thoracic artery
Temporal artery	Middle temporal artery, Superficial temporal artery, Transverse facial artery
Thyroid artery	Cricothyroid artery, Hyoid artery, Sternocleidomastoid artery, Superior laryngeal artery, Superior thyroid artery, Thyrocervical trunk
Ulnar artery	Anterior ulnar recurrent artery, Common interosseous artery, Posterior ulnar recurrent artery
Vertebral artery	Anterior spinal artery, Posterior spinal artery

Table 2.5   Lower Arteries Body Part key by ICD-10-PCS description

ICD-10-PCS Term	Anatomical Term(s)
Abdominal aorta	Inferior phrenic artery, Lumbar artery, Median sacral artery, Middle suprarenal artery, Ovarian artery, Testicular artery
Anterior tibial artery	Anterior lateral malleolar artery, Anterior medial malleolar artery, Anterior tibial recurrent artery, Dorsalis pedis artery, Posterior tibial recurrent artery
Celiac artery	Celiac trunk
External iliac artery	Deep circumflex iliac artery, Inferior epigastric artery
Femoral artery	Circumflex iliac artery, Deep femoral artery, Descending genicular artery, External pudendal artery, Superficial epigastric artery
Foot artery	Arcuate artery, Dorsal metatarsal artery, Lateral plantar artery, Lateral tarsal artery, Medial plantar artery
Gastric artery	Left gastric artery, Right gastric artery
Hepatic artery	Common hepatic artery, Gastroduodenal artery, Hepatic artery proper
Inferior mesenteric artery	Sigmoid artery, Superior rectal artery
Internal iliac artery	Deferential artery, Hypogastric artery, Iliolumbar artery, Inferior gluteal artery, Inferior vesical artery, Internal pudendal artery, Lateral sacral artery, Middle rectal artery, Obturator artery, Superior gluteal artery, Umbilical artery, Uterine artery, Vaginal artery
Peroneal artery	Fibular artery
Popliteal artery	Inferior genicular artery, Middle genicular artery, Superior genicular artery, Sural artery
Renal artery	Inferior suprarenal artery, Renal segmental artery
Splenic artery	Left gastroepiploic artery, Pancreatic artery, Short gastric artery
Superior mesenteric artery	Ileal artery, Ileocolic artery, Inferior pancreaticoduodenal artery, Jejunal artery

Table 2.6   Upper Veins Body Part key by ICD-10-PCS description

ICD-10-PCS Term	Anatomical Term(s)
Azygos vein	Right ascending lumbar vein, Right subcostal vein
Basilic vein	Median antebrachial vein, Median cubital vein
Brachial vein	Radial vein, Ulnar vein
Cephalic vein	Accessory cephalic vein
External jugular vein	Posterior auricular vein
Face vein	Angular vein, Anterior facial vein, Common facial vein, Deep facial vein, Frontal vein, Posterior facial (retromandibular) vein, Supraorbital vein
Hand vein	Dorsal metacarpal vein, Palmar (volar) metacarpal vein, Palmar (volar) digital vein, Superficial palmar venous arch, Volar (palmar) metacarpal vein, Volar (palmar) digital vein
Hemiazygos vein	Left ascending lumbar vein, Left subcostal vein
Innominate vein	Brachiocephalic vein, Inferior thyroid vein
Intracranial vein	Anterior cerebral vein, Basal (internal) cerebral vein, Dural venous sinus, Great cerebral vein, Inferior cerebral vein, Inferior cerebellar vein, Internal (basal) cerebral vein, Middle cerebral vein, Ophthalmic vein, Superior cerebral vein, Superior cerebellar vein
Vertebral vein	Deep cervical vein, Suboccipital venous plexus

Table 2.7   Lower Veins Body Part key by ICD-10-PCS description

ICD-10-PCS Term	Anatomical Term(s)
Colic vein	Ileocolic vein, Left colic vein, Middle colic vein, Right colic vein
Femoral vein	Deep femoral (profunda femoris) vein, Popliteal vein, Profunda femoris (deep femoral) vein
Foot vein	Common digital vein, Dorsal metatarsal vein, Dorsal venous arch, Plantar digital vein, Plantar metatarsal vein, Plantar venous arch
Greater saphenous vein	External pudendal vein, Great saphenous vein, Superficial epigastric vein, Superficial circumflex iliac vein
Hypogastric vein	Gluteal vein, Internal iliac vein, Internal pudendal vein, Lateral sacral vein, Middle hemorrhoidal vein, Obturator vein, Uterine vein, Vaginal vein, Vesical vein
Inferior mesenteric vein	Sigmoid vein, Superior rectal vein
Inferior vena cava	Postcava, Right inferior phrenic vein, Right ovarian vein, Right second lumbar vein, Right suprarenal vein, Right testicular vein
Lesser saphenous vein	Small saphenous vein
Portal vein	Hepatic portal vein
Renal vein, left	Left inferior phrenic vein, Left ovarian vein, Left second lumbar vein, Left suprarenal vein, Left testicular vein
Splenic vein	Left gastroepiploic vein, Pancreatic vein
Superior mesenteric vein	Right gastroepiploic vein

Lymphatic and Hemic Systems

In ICD-10-PCS, the structures of the lymphatic and hemic systems affecting procedural code assignment include the following: lymphatic, head; lymphatic, neck; lymphatic, upper extremity; lymphatic, axillary; lymphatic, thorax; lymphatic, internal mammary; lymphatic, mesenteric; lymphatic, pelvis; lymphatic, aortic; lymphatic, lower extremity; lymphatic, inguinal, thoracic duct, cisternal chyli, thymus; lymphatic, spleen, bone marrow, sternum, bone marrow, iliac, bone marrow vertebral, bone marrow.

The lymphatic system is a network of conduits that carry lymph and lymphatic tissue and vessels. The lymphatic system is a one-way system in which the lymph flows toward the heart. Many organs contain lymphoid tissue such as lymph nodes, spleen, tonsils and adenoids, and the thymus. This lymphatic tissue is concerned with immune functions in defending the body against infections and spread of tumors.

A lymph node is a collection of lymphoid tissue located at intervals along the lymphatic system. Clusters of lymph nodes are found in the axilla, groin, neck, and abdomen.

The lymphatic system consists of afferent lymph vessels which bring in lymph to the lymph node and then is drained out by the efferent lymph vessel. The outer part of the lymph node is the cortex and the inner portion is called the medulla.

In ICD-10-PCS to code some root operations it is necessary to know if a lymph node, lymph nodes, or lymph node chain is excised. The National Cancer Institute's SEER training modules have references on lymph node chains. See http://training.seer.cancer.gov/lymphoma/anatomy/chains/.

ICD-10-PCS Body Part Key

The ICD-10-PCS terms used to describe a body part may correspond to anatomical terms. To bridge the two, consult table 2.8.

Table 2.8   Lymphatic and Hemic Systems Body Part key by ICD-10-PCS description

ICD-10-PCS Term	Anatomical Term(s)
Cisterna chyli	Intestinal lymphatic trunk, Lumbar lymphatic trunk
Lymphatic, aortic	Celiac lymph node, Gastric lymph node, Hepatic lymph node, Lumbar lymph node, Pancreaticosplenic lymph node, Para-aortic lymph node, Retroperitoneal lymph node
Lymphatic, axillary	Anterior (pectoral) lymph node, Apical (subclavicular) lymph node, Brachial (lateral) lymph node, Central axillary lymph node, Lateral (brachial) lymph node, Pectoral (anterior) lymph node, Posterior (subscapular) lymph node, Subclavicular (apical) lymph node, Subscapular (posterior) lymph node
Lymphatic, head	Buccinator lymph node, Infra-auricular lymph node, Infraparotid lymph node, Parotid lymph node, Preauricular lymph node, Submandibular lymph node, Submaxillary lymph node, Submental lymph node, Subparotid lymph node, Suprahyoid lymph node
Lymphatic, lower extremity	Femoral lymph node, Popliteal lymph node
Lymphatic, mesenteric	Inferior mesenteric lymph node, Pararectal lymph node, Superior mesenteric lymph node
Lymphatic, neck	Cervical lymph node, Jugular lymph node, Mastoid (post-auricular) lymph node, Occipital lymph node, Postauricular (mastoid) lymph node, Retropharyngeal lymph node, Supraclavicular (Virchow's) lymph node (left), Virchow's (supraclavicular) lymph node (left), Right jugular trunk, Right lymphatic duct, Right subclavian trunk
Lymphatic, pelvis	Common iliac (subaortic) lymph node, Gluteal lymph node, Iliac lymph node, Inferior epigastric lymph node, Obturator lymph node, Sacral lymph node, Subaortic (common iliac) lymph node, Suprainguinal lymph node
Lymphatic, thorax	Intercostal lymph node, Mediastinal lymph node, Parasternal lymph node, Paratracheal lymph node, Tracheobronchial lymph node
Lymphatic, upper extremity	Cubital lymph node, Deltopectoral (infraclavicular) lymph node, Epitrochlear lymph node, Infraclavicular (deltopectoral) lymph node, Supratrochlear lymph node
Spleen	Accessory spleen
Thoracic duct	Left jugular trunk, Left subclavian trunk
Thymus	Thymus gland

Eye

In ICD-10-PCS, the structures of the eye affecting procedural code assignment include the following: eye, anterior chamber, vitreous, sclera, cornea, choroid, iris, retina, retinal vessel, lens, extraocular muscle, eyelid (upper and lower), conjunctiva, lacrimal gland, and lacrimal duct. All body parts have a left or right designation. If a bilateral procedure is performed, then two codes would be assigned.

The structures of the eye include the vitreous, which is often referred to as the vitreous body or vitreous humor. It is contained in a thin hyoid membrane and consists of a transparent, semigelatinous substance that fills the cavity behind the crystalline lens of the eye and in front of the retina. Blood vessels which supply and drain the retina include the central retinal artery and its branches along with the central retinal vein and its branches.

The oculomotor muscles are the medial rectus, lateral rectus, superior rectus, inferior rectus, inferior oblique, superior oblique, musculus orbitalis, and levator palpebrae superioris. The orbitalis muscle is also known as the orbital muscle of Müller.

The lacrimal (tear) gland and duct (excretory duct of lacrimal gland) are part of the lacrimal apparatus, a tear-forming and tear-conducting system. The lacrimal gland is located above and lateral to the eye in the orbit. Located in each eyelid, other names for the lacrimal duct are lacrimal canaliculi or lacrimal canals. The nasolacrimal duct extends from the lacrimal sac to the inferior meatus of the nose.

ICD-10-PCS Body Part Key

The ICD-10-PCS terms used to describe a body part may correspond to anatomical terms. To bridge the two, consult table 2.9.

Table 2.9.   Eye Body Part key by ICD-10-PCS description

ICD-10-PCS Term	Anatomical Term(s)
Anterior chamber	Aqueous humour
Conjunctiva	Plica semilunaris
Extraocular muscle	Inferior oblique, Inferior rectus, Lateral rectus, Medial rectus, Superior oblique, Superior rectus
Eye	Ciliary body, posterior chamber
Lacrimal duct	Lacrimal canaliculus, Lacrimal punctum, Lacrimal sac, Nasolacrimal duct
Lens	Zonule of Zinn
Retina	Fovea, Macula, Optic disc
Vitreous	Vitreous body

Ear, Nose, Sinus

In ICD-10-PCS, the structures of the ear, nose, and sinus affecting procedural code assignment include the following: external ear, auditory canal, middle ear, tympanic membrane, auditory ossicle, mastoid sinus, inner ear, Eustachian tube, ear, nose, nasal turbinate, nasal septum, nasopharynx, accessory sinus, maxillary sinus, frontal sinus, ethmoid sinus, sphenoid sinus, and sinus.

The external or outer ear includes the pinna and ear lobe along with the external auditory canal which leads to the tympanic membrane or eardrum. Components of the middle ear are the eardrum, ossicles or ear bones, and the air cells behind the eardrum in the mastoid cavities. The ossicles are the hammer (malleus), anvil (incus) and stirrup (stapes). Located within the temporal bone, the semicircular canals, vestibule, and cochlea comprise the inner (internal) ear. The inner ear is sometimes referred to as the labyrinth.

The four paranasal or accessory sinuses are listed in table 2.10. These cavities are found inside the bones near the nose. Their names reflect the bone in which the sinus is found.

ICD-10-PCS Body Part Key

The ICD-10-PCS terms used to describe a body part may correspond to anatomical terms. To bridge the two, consult table 2.11.

Table 2.10. Paranasal Sinuses by ICD-10-PCS description

ICD-10-PCS Name	Location
Ethmoid	Within the ethmoid bone between the nose and the eyes
Frontal	Within the frontal bone beneath the forehead
Maxillary	Within the maxillary bone under the eye
Sphenoid	Within the sphenoid bone at the center of the skull base under the pituitary gland

Table 2.11 Ear, Nose, and Sinus Body Part key by ICD-10-PCS description

ICD-10-PCS Term	Anatomical Term(s)
Auditory ossicle	Incus, Malleus, Ossicular chain, Stapes
Ethmoid sinus	Ethmoidal air cell
Eustachian tube	Auditory tube, Pharyngotympanic tube
External auditory canal	External auditory meatus
External ear	Antihelix, Antitragus, Auricle, Earlobe, Helix, Pinna, Tragus
Inner ear	Bony labyrinth, Bony vestibule, Cochlea, Oval window, Round window, Semicircular canal
Mastoid sinus	Mastoid air cells
Maxillary sinus	Antrum of Highmore
Middle ear	Tympanic cavity
Nasal septum	Quadrangular cartilage, Septal cartilage, Vomer
Nasal turbinate	Inferior turbinate, Middle turbinate, Nasal concha, Superior turbinate
Nasopharynx	Choana, Fossa of Rosenmuller, Pharyngeal recess, Rhinopharynx
Tympanic membrane	Pars flaccida

Respiratory System

In ICD-10-PCS, the structures of the respiratory system affecting procedural code assignment include the following portions of this system: tracheobronchial tree, trachea, carina, bronchus (main, upper lobe, middle lobe, lower lobe, lingula), lung (lower lobe, upper lobe, middle lobe, lingual), lung, pleura, and diaphragm.

The organs and structures of the respiratory system include the tracheobronchial tree—the trachea, bronchi, and bronchioles. A ridge at the base of the trachea that separates the openings of the right and left main bronchi is called the carina tracheae.

Pleura is a membrane consisting of two large thin layers of tissue, one that wraps around the outside of the lungs, and another that lines the inside of the chest cavity. There is a thin space between the layers and the pleura (pleural space) that is filled with a small amount of fluid that enables the layers of the pleura to glide smoothly during breathing.

During breathing, air enters the nose or mouth and moves to the trachea, which splits into the bronchial tubes that enter the lungs. The lungs allow oxygen exchange as previously discussed in the circulatory system. The bronchi branch into thousands of smaller, thinner tubes called bronchioles which end in bunches of round air sacs called alveoli. The alveoli are covered by a mesh of capillaries.

There is no applicable body part key for this system, as the body part values are represented in ICD-10-PCS.

Mouth and Throat

In ICD-10-PCS, the structures of the mouth and throat affecting procedural code assignment include the following: lip (upper and lower), palate (hard and soft), buccal mucosa, gingiva (upper and lower), tongue, parotid gland, salivary gland, parotid duct, sublingual gland, submaxillary (submandibular) gland, minor salivary gland, pharynx, uvula, tonsils, adenoids, epiglottis, larynx, vocal cord, tooth (upper and lower), and the generic "mouth and throat." The larynx consists of three main parts:

- Supraglottis (top part)
- Glottis (middle part containing vocal cords)
- Subglottic (bottom part that connects the trachea)

The pharynx is divided into three sections: The nasopharynx, oropharynx, and laryngopharynx (hypopharynx).

ICD-10-PCS Body Part Key

The ICD-10-PCS terms used to describe a body part may correspond to anatomical terms. To bridge the two, consult table 2.12.

Table 2.12.   Mouth and Throat Body Part key by ICD-10-PCS description

ICD-10-PCS Term	Anatomical Term(s)
Adenoids	Pharyngeal tonsil
Buccal Mucosa	Buccal gland, Labial gland, Molar gland, Palatine gland
Epiglottis	Glossoepiglottic fold
Larynx	Aryepiglottic fold, Arytenoid cartilage, Corniculate cartilage, Cricoid cartilage, Cuneiform cartilage, False vocal cord, Glottis, Rima glottidis, Thyroid cartilage, Ventricular fold
Lower Lip	Frenulum labii inferioris, Vermilion border
Minor Salivary Gland	Anterior lingual gland
Parotid Duct	Stensen's duct
Pharynx	Hypopharynx, Laryngopharynx, Oropharynx, Piriform recess (sinus)
Submaxillary Gland	Submandibular gland
Tongue	Frenulum linguae, Lingual tonsil
Tonsils	Palatine tonsil
Upper Lip	Frenulum labii superioris, Vermilion border
Uvula	Palatine uvula
Vocal Cord	Vocal fold

Gastrointestinal

In ICD-10-PCS, the structures of the digestive system affecting procedural code assignment include the following portions of this system:
upper intestinal tract, esophagus (upper, middle, lower), esophagogastric junction, esophagus, stomach, pylorus, small intestine, duodenum,
jejunum, ileum, ileocecal valve, lower intestinal tract, large intestine,
cecum, appendix, ascending colon, transverse colon, descending colon,
sigmoid colon, rectum, anus, anal sphincter, omentum (greater and
lesser), mesentery, and peritoneum.

ICD-10-PCS Body Part Key

The ICD-10-PCS terms used to describe a body part may correspond to
anatomical terms. To bridge the two, consult table 2.13.

**Table 2.13.   Gastrointestinal System Body Part key by ICD-10-PCS
description**

ICD-10-PCS Term	Anatomical Term(s)
Anus	Anal orifice
Appendix	Vermiform appendix
Ascending Colon	Hepatic flexure
Esophagogastric Junction	Cardia, Cardioesophageal junction, Gastroesophageal (GE) junction
Esophagus, Lower	Abdominal esophagus
Esophagus, Middle	Thoracic esophagus
Esophagus, Upper	Cervical esophagus
Greater Omentum	Gastrocolic omentum, Gastrocolic ligament, Gastrophrenic ligament, Gastrosplenic ligament
Jejunum	Duodenojejunal flexure
Lesser Omentum	Gastrohepatic omentum, Hepatogastric ligament
Mesentery	Mesoappendix, Mesocolon
Peritoneum	Epiploic foramen

Table 2.13.   (Continued)

ICD-10-PCS Term	Anatomical Term(s)
Rectum	Anorectal junction
Sigmoid Colon	Rectosigmoid junction, Sigmoid flexure
Stomach, Pylorus	Pyloric antrum, Pyloric canal, Pyloric sphincter
Transverse Colon	Splenic flexure

Hepatobiliary System and Pancreas

In ICD-10-PCS, the structures of the hepatobiliary system and pancreas affecting procedural code assignment include the following: liver (right and left lobe), gallbladder, hepatic duct, cystic duct, common bile duct, hepatobiliary duct, ampulla of Vater, pancreatic duct, accessory pancreatic duct, and pancreas.

Hepatobiliary refers to the liver and bile ducts. Bile ducts are channels that collect and transport the bile secretion from the bile canaliculi, the smallest branch of the biliary tract in the liver, through the bile ductules, the bile ducts out the liver, and to the gallbladder for storage (NLM n.d.).

ICD-10-PCS Body Part Key

The ICD-10-PCS terms used to describe a body part may correspond to anatomical terms. To bridge the two, consult table 2.14.

Table 2.14.   Hepatobiliary System and Pancreas Body Part key by ICD-10-PCS description

ICD-10-PCS Term	Anatomical Term(s)
Ampulla of Vater	Duodenal ampulla, Hepatopancreatic ampulla
Liver	Quadrate lobe
Pancreatic Duct, Accessory	Duct of Santorini
Pancreatic Duct	Duct of Wirsung

Endocrine System

In ICD-10-PCS, the structures of the endocrine system affecting procedural code assignment include the following portions of this system: pituitary gland, pineal body, adrenal gland, carotid body, para-aortic body, coccygeal glomus, glomus jugulare, aortic body, paraganglion extremity, thyroid gland, thyroid gland isthmus, superior parathyroid gland, inferior parathyroid gland, and the generic "endocrine gland."

The endocrine glands consist of the pituitary, pineal, thyroid and parathyroids, adrenals, the islets of Langerhans found in the pancreas, gonads found in the testes and ovaries.

The organs that secrete hormones are found in other sections of ICD-10-PCS. These include:

- The hypothalamus—central nervous system
- The pancreas—hepatobiliary system
- The ovaries—female reproductive system
- The testes—male reproductive system

It is necessary to know the location of the thyroid gland, including the isthmus and the parathyroid gland.

Other body parts, their synonyms, and location are described in table 2.15.

Table 2.15. Endocrine Body Part, synonyms, and location

ICD-10-PCS Name	Other Names	Location
Pituitary gland	Hypophysis	Brain
Pineal body	Pineal gland, Epiphysis cerebri, Epiphysis or the "third eye"	Brain
Parathyroid Superior Inferior	Parathyroid IVs Parathyroid IIIs	Neck Usually at the middle of the posterior border of the thyroid lobe Usually near the lower pole of the thyroid gland
Adrenal	Suprarenal glands	Top of each kidney
Carotid body	Carotid, glomus, Glomus caroticum, Glomus caroticus	Paraganglia structure located near the bifurcation of the internal carotid artery

Table 2.15.   (Continued)

ICD-10-PCS Name	Other Names	Location
Para-Aortic body	Organ of Zuckerkandl, Aortic glomera, Corpora paraaortica, Body of Zuckerkandl	Paraganglia structure found near the sympathetic ganglia along the abdominal aorta, beginning cranial to the superior mesenteric artery or renal arteries and extending to the level of the aortic bifurcation or just beyond
Coccygeal glomus	Glomus coccygeum, Coccygeal gland or body; Luschka's gland or body	Paraganglia structure in front of, or immediately below, the tip of the coccyx
Glomus Jugulare		Paraganglia structure in the wall of the jugular bulb
Aortic body	Aortic glomus, Glomus aorticum, Vagal body, Aortic ganglion	Paraganglia structure near the arch of the aorta, the pulmonary arteries, and the coronary arteries
Paraganglion extremity		Paraganglia structure found along the iliac and femoral vessels particularly the around the *iliac* bifurcation

ICD-10-PCS Body Part Key

The ICD-10-PCS terms used to describe a body part may correspond to anatomical terms. To bridge the two, consult table 2.16.

Table 2.16.   Endocrine System Body Part key by ICD-10-PCS description

ICD-10-PCS Term	Anatomical Term(s)
Adrenal gland	Suprarenal gland
Carotid body	Carotid glomus
Coccygeal Glomus	Coccygeal body
Glomus Jugulare	Jugular body
Pituitary gland	Adenohypophysis, Hypophysis, Neurohypophysis

Musculoskeletal System

In ICD-10-PCS, the general structures of the musculoskeletal system affecting procedural code assignment include the following: muscles, tendons, bursa, ligaments, bones, and joints.

In ICD-10-PCS, the structures of the muscles affecting procedural code assignment include the following: head, facial, neck, tongue, palate and pharynx, shoulder, upper arm, lower arm and wrist, hand, trunk, thorax, abdomen, perineum, hip, upper leg, lower leg, foot, and upper and lower muscle.

In ICD-10-PCS, the structures of the tendons affecting procedural code assignment include the following: head and neck, shoulder, upper arm, lower arm and wrist, hand, trunk, thorax, abdomen, perineum, hip, upper leg, lower leg, knee, ankle, foot, and upper and lower tendon.

In ICD-10-PCS, the structures of the bursae and ligaments affecting procedural code assignment include the following: head and neck, shoulder, elbow, wrist, hand, upper extremity, trunk, thorax, abdomen, perineum, hip, knee, ankle, foot, lower extremity, and upper and lower bursa and ligament.

In ICD-10-PCS, the structures of the head and facial bones affecting procedural code assignment include the following: skull, frontal, parietal, temporal, occipital, nasal, sphenoid, ethmoid, lacrimal, palatine, zygomatic, orbit, maxilla, mandible, facial, and hyoid bones.

In ICD-10-PCS, the structures of the upper bones affecting procedural code assignment include the following: sternum, rib, cervical vertebra, thoracic vertebra, scapula, glenoid cavity, clavicle, humeral head, humeral shaft, radius, ulna, carpal, metacarpal, thumb phalanx, finger phalanx, and upper bone.

In ICD-10-PCS, the structures of the lower bones affecting procedural code assignment include the following: lumbar vertebra, sacrum, pelvic, acetabulum, upper femur, femoral shaft, lower femur, patella, tibia, fibula, tarsal, metatarsal, toe phalanx, coccyx, and lower bone.

In ICD-10-PCS, the structures of the upper joints affecting procedural code assignment include the following: occipital-cervical, cervical vertebral, cervicothoracic vertebral, thoracic vertebral, thoracolumbar vertebral, temporomandibular, sternoclavicular, acromioclavicular, shoulder, elbow, wrist, carpal, metacarpocarpal, metacarpophalangeal, finger phalangeal, upper joints and cervical vertebral, cervicothoracic vertebral, thoracic vertebral, and thoracolumbar vertebral discs.

In ICD-10-PCS, the structures of the lower joints affecting procedural code assignment include the following: lumbar vertebral, lumbosacral, sacrococcygeal, coccygeal, sacroiliac, hip, knee, ankle, tarsal, metatarsal-tarsal, metatarsal-phalangeal, toe phalangeal, and lower joints and lumbar vertebral, and lumbosacral discs.

ICD-10-PCS Body Part Key

The ICD-10-PCS terms used to describe a body part may correspond to anatomical terms. To bridge the two, consult tables 2.17–2.24.

Table 2.17.   Muscle Body Part key by ICD-10-PCS description

ICD-10-PCS Term	Anatomical Term(s)
Abdomen Muscle	External oblique muscle, Internal oblique muscle, Pyramidalis muscle, Rectus abdominis muscle, Transversus abdominis muscle
Facial Muscle	Buccinator muscle, Corrugator supercilii muscle, Depressor anguli oris muscle, Depressor labii inferioris muscle, Depressor septi nasi muscle, Depressor supercilii muscle, Levator anguli oris muscle, Levator labii superioris muscle, Levator labii superioris alaeque nasi muscle, Mentalis muscle, Nasalis muscle, Occipitofrontalis muscle, Orbicularis oris muscle, Procerus muscle, Risorius muscle, Zygomaticus muscle
Foot Muscle	Abductor hallucis muscle, Adductor hallucis muscle, Extensor digitorum brevis muscle, Extensor hallucis brevis muscle, Flexor digitorum brevis muscle, Flexor hallucis brevis muscle, Quadratus plantae muscle
Hand Muscle	Hypothenar muscle, Palmar interosseous muscle, Thenar muscle
Head Muscle	Auricularis muscle, Masseter muscle, Pterygoid muscle, Splenius capitis muscle, Temporalis muscle, Temporoparietalis muscle
Hip Muscle	Gemellus muscle, Gluteus maximus muscle, Gluteus medius muscle, Gluteus minimus muscle, Iliacus muscle, Obturator muscle, Piriformis muscle, Psoas muscle, Quadratus femoris muscle, Tensor fasciae latae muscle
Lower Arm and Wrist Muscle	Brachioradialis muscle, Extensor carpi ulnaris muscle, Extensor carpi radialis muscle, Flexor carpi ulnaris muscle, Flexor carpi radialis muscle, Flexor pollicis longus muscle, Palmaris longus muscle, Pronator quadratus muscle, Pronator teres muscle
Lower Leg Muscle	Extensor digitorum longus muscle, Extensor hallucis longus muscle, Fibularis brevis muscle, Fibularis longus muscle, Flexor digitorum longus muscle, Flexor hallucis longus muscle, Gastrocnemius muscle, Peroneus brevis muscle, Peroneus longus muscle, Popliteus muscle, Soleus muscle, Tibialis anterior muscle, Tibialis posterior muscle

(Continued on next page)

Table 2.17. (Continued)

ICD-10-PCS Term	Anatomical Term(s)
Neck Muscle	Anterior vertebral muscle, Arytenoid muscle, Cricothyroid muscle, Infrahyoid muscle, Levator scapulae muscle, Platysma muscle, Scalene muscle, Splenius cervicis muscle, Sternocleidomastoid muscle, Suprahyoid muscle, Thyroarytenoid muscle
Perineum Muscle	Bulbospongiosus muscle, Cremaster muscle, Deep transverse perineal muscle, Ischiocavernosus muscle, Superficial transverse perineal muscle
Shoulder Muscle	Deltoid muscle, Infraspinatus muscle, Subscapularis muscle, Supraspinatus muscle, Teres major muscle, Teres minor muscle
Thorax Muscle	Intercostal muscle, Levatores costarum muscle, Pectoralis minor muscle, Pectoralis major muscle, Serratus anterior muscle, Subclavius muscle, Subcostal muscle, Transverse thoracis muscle
Tongue, Palate, Pharynx Muscle	Chondroglossus muscle, Genioglossus muscle, Hyoglossus muscle, Inferior longitudinal muscle, Levator veli palatini muscle, Palatoglossal muscle, Palatopharyngeal muscle, Pharyngeal constrictor muscle, Salpingopharyngeus muscle, Styloglossus muscle, Stylopharyngeus muscle, Superior longitudinal muscle, Tensor veli palatini muscle
Trunk Muscle	Coccygeus muscle, Erector spinae muscle, Interspinalis muscle, Intertransversarius muscle, Latissimus dorsi muscle, Levator ani muscle, Quadratus lumborum muscle, Rhomboid major muscle, Rhomboid minor muscle, Serratus posterior muscle, Transversospinalis muscle, Trapezius muscle
Upper Arm Muscle	Biceps brachii muscle, Brachialis muscle, Coracobrachialis muscle, Triceps brachii muscle
Upper Leg Muscle	Adductor brevis muscle, Adductor longus muscle, Adductor magnus muscle, Biceps femoris muscle, Gracilis muscle, Pectineus muscle, Quadriceps (femoris), Rectus femoris muscle, Sartorius muscle, Semimembranosus muscle, Semitendinosus muscle, Vastus intermedius muscle, Vastus lateralis muscle, Vastus medialis muscle

A tendon is a tough band of fibrous connective tissue that usually connects muscle to bone. Tendons are similar to ligaments and fascia—both are made of collagen—except that ligaments join one bone to another bone, and fascia connect muscles to other muscles.

Table 2.18. Tendon Body Part key by ICD-10-PCS description

ICD-10-PCS Term	Anatomical Term(s)
Abdomen Tendon	External oblique tendon, Internal oblique tendon, Pyramidalis tendon, Rectus abdominis tendon, Transversus abdominis tendon
Foot Tendon	Abductor hallucis tendon, Adductor hallucis tendon, Extensor digitorum brevis tendon, Extensor hallucis brevis tendon, Flexor digitorum brevis tendon, Flexor hallucis brevis tendon, Quadratus plantae tendon
Hand Tendon	Hypothenar tendon, Palmar interosseous tendon, Thenar tendon
Head and Neck Tendon	Anterior vertebral tendon, Arytenoid tendon, Auricularis tendon, Cricothyroid tendon, Infrahyoid tendon, Levator scapulae tendon, Masseter tendon, Platysma tendon, Pterygoid tendon, Scalene tendon, Splenius capitis tendon, Splenius cervicis tendon, Sternocleidomastoid tendon, Suprahyoid tendon, Temporalis tendon, Temporoparietalis tendon, Thyroarytenoid tendon
Hip Tendon	Gemellus tendon, Gluteus maximus tendon, Gluteus medius tendon, Gluteus minimus tendon, Iliacus tendon, Obturator tendon, Piriformis tendon, Psoas tendon, Quadratus femoris tendon, Tensor fasciae latae tendon
Knee Tendon	Patellar tendon
Lower Arm and Wrist Tendon	Anatomical snuffbox, Brachioradialis tendon, Extensor carpi ulnaris tendon, Extensor carpi radialis tendon, Flexor carpi ulnaris tendon, Flexor carpi radialis tendon, Flexor pollicis longus tendon, Palmaris longus tendon, Pronator quadrates tendon, Pronator teres tendon
Lower Leg Tendon	Achilles tendon, Extensor digitorum longus tendon, Extensor hallucis longus tendon, Fibularis brevis tendon, Fibularis longus tendon, Flexor digitorum longus tendon, Flexor hallucis longus tendon, Gastrocnemius tendon, Peroneus brevis tendon, Peroneus longus tendon, Popliteus tendon, Soleus tendon, Tibialis anterior tendon, Tibialis posterior tendon
Perineum Tendon	Bulbospongiosus tendon, Cremaster tendon, Deep transverse perineal tendon, Ischiocavernosus tendon, Superficial transverse perineal tendon

(Continued on next page)

Table 2.18.   (Continued)

ICD-10-PCS Term	Anatomical Term(s)
Shoulder Tendon	Deltoid tendon, Infraspinatus tendon, Subscapularis tendon, Supraspinatus tendon, Teres major tendon, Teres minor tendon
Thorax Tendon	Intercostal tendon, Levatores costarum tendon, Pectoralis minor tendon, Pectoralis major tendon, Serratus anterior tendon, Subclavius tendon, Subcostal tendon, Transverse thoracis tendon
Trunk Tendon	Coccygeus tendon, Erector spinae tendon, Interspinalis tendon, Intertransversarius tendon, Latissimus dorsi tendon, Levator ani tendon, Quadratus lumborum tendon, Rhomboid major tendon, Rhomboid minor tendon, Serratus posterior tendon, Transversospinalis tendon, Trapezius tendon
Upper Arm Tendon	Biceps brachii tendon, Brachialis tendon, Coraco-brachialis tendon, Triceps brachii tendon
Upper Leg Tendon	Adductor brevis tendon, Adductor longus tendon, Adductor magnus tendon, Biceps femoris tendon, Gracilis tendon, Pectineus tendon, Quadriceps (femoris), Rectus femoris tendon, Sartorius tendon, Semimembranosus tendon, Semitendinosus tendon, Vastus intermedius tendon, Vastus lateralis tendon, Vastus medialis tendon

Bursae, flat, fluid-filled sacs found between a bone and a tendon or muscle, form a cushion to help the tendon or muscle slide smoothly over the bone. Ligaments are shiny, flexible bands of fibrous tissue connecting together articular extremities of bones.

Table 2.19.   Bursa and Ligament Body Part key by ICD-10-PCS description

ICD-10-PCS Term	Anatomical Term(s)
Ankle Bursa and Ligament	Calcaneofibular ligament, Deltoid ligament, Ligament of the lateral malleolus, Talofibular ligament
Elbow Bursa and Ligament	Annular ligament, Olecranon bursa, Radial collateral ligament, Ulnar collateral ligament

Table 2.19.   (Continued)

ICD-10-PCS Term	Anatomical Term(s)
Foot Bursa and Ligament	Calcaneocuboid ligament, Cuneonavicular ligament, Intercuneiform ligament, Interphalangeal ligament, Metatarsal ligament, Metatarsophalangeal ligament, Subtalar ligament, Talocalcaneal ligament, Talocalcaneonavicular ligament, Tarsometatarsal ligament
Hand Bursa and Ligament	Carpometacarpal ligament, Intercarpal ligament, Interphalangeal ligament, Lunotriquetral ligament, Metacarpal ligament, Metacarpophalangeal ligament, Pisohamate ligament, Pisometacarpal ligament, Scapholunate ligament, Scaphotrapezium ligament
Head and Neck Bursa and Ligament	Alar ligament of axis, Cervical intertransverse ligament, Cervical interspinous ligament, Cervical ligamentum flavum, Lateral temporomandibular ligament, Sphenomandibular ligament, Stylomandibular ligament, Transverse ligament of atlas
Hip Bursa and Ligament	Iliofemoral ligament, Ischiofemoral ligament, Pubofemoral ligament, Transverse acetabular ligament, Trochanteric bursa
Knee Bursa and Ligament	Anterior cruciate ligament (ACL), Lateral collateral ligament (LCL), Ligament of head of fibula, Medial collateral ligament (MCL), Patellar ligament, Popliteal ligament, Posterior cruciate ligament (PCL), Prepatellar bursa
Shoulder Bursa and Ligament	Acromioclavicular ligament, Coracoacromial ligament, Coracoclavicular ligament, Coracohumeral ligament, Costoclavicular ligament, Glenohumeral ligament, Glenoid ligament (labrum), Interclavicular ligament, Sternoclavicular ligament, Subacromial bursa, Transverse humeral ligament, Transverse scapular ligament
Thorax Bursa and Ligament	Costotransverse ligament, Costoxiphoid ligament, Sternocostal ligament
Trunk Bursa and Ligament	Iliolumbar ligament, Interspinous ligament, Intertransverse ligament, Ligamentum flavum, Pubic ligament, Sacrococcygeal ligament, Sacroiliac ligament, Sacrospinous ligament, Sacrotuberous ligament, Supraspinous ligament
Wrist Bursa and Ligament	Palmar ulnocarpal ligament, Radial collateral carpal ligament, Radiocarpal ligament, Radioulnar ligament, Ulnar collateral carpal ligament

Table 2.20.   Head and Facial Bones Body Part key by ICD-10-PCS description

ICD-10-PCS Term	Anatomical Term(s)
Ethmoid Bone	Cribriform plate
Frontal Bone	Zygomatic process of frontal bone
Mandible	Alveolar process of mandible, Condyloid process, Mandibular notch, Mental foramen
Maxilla	Alveolar process of maxilla
Nasal Bone	Vomer
Occipital Bone	Foramen magnum
Orbit	Bony orbit, Orbital portion of zygomatic bone, Orbital portion of sphenoid bone, Orbital portion of palatine bone, Orbital portion of maxilla, Orbital portion of lacrimal bone, Orbital portion of frontal bone, Orbital portion of ethmoid bone
Sphenoid Bone	Greater wing, Lesser wing, Optic foramen, Pterygoid process, Sella turcica
Temporal Bone	Mastoid process, Petrous part of temporal bone, Tympanic part of temporal bone, Zygomatic process of temporal bone

Table 2.21.   Upper Bones Body Part key by ICD-10-PCS description

ICD-10-PCS Term	Anatomical Term(s)
Carpal	Capitate bone, Hamate bone, Lunate bone, Pisiform bone, Scaphoid bone, Trapezium bone, Trapezoid bone, Triquetral bone
Cervical Vertebra	Spinous process, Vertebral arch, Vertebral foramen, Vertebral lamina, Vertebral pedicle
Glenoid Cavity	Glenoid fossa (of scapula)
Humeral Head	Greater tuberosity, Lesser tuberosity, Neck of humerus (anatomical)(surgical)

Table 2.21. (Continued)

ICD-10-PCS Term	Anatomical Term(s)
Humeral Shaft	Lateral epicondyle of humerus, Medial epicondyle of humerus
Radius	Ulnar notch
Scapula	Acromion (process), Coracoid process
Sternum	Manubrium, Suprasternal notch, Xiphoid process
Thoracic Vertebra	Spinous process, Vertebral arch, Vertebral foramen, Vertebral lamina, Vertebral pedicle
Ulna	Olecranon process, Radial notch

Table 2.22 Lower Bones Body Part key by ICD-10-PCS description

ICD-10-PCS Term	Anatomical Term(s)
Femoral Shaft	Body of femur
Fibula	Body of fibula, Head of fibula, Lateral malleolus
Lower Femur	Lateral condyle of femur, Lateral epicondyle of femur, Medial condyle of femur, Medial epicondyle of femur
Lumbar Vertebra	Spinous process, Vertebral arch, Vertebral foramen, Vertebral lamina, Vertebral pedicle
Pelvic Bone	Iliac crest, Ilium, Ischium, Pubis
Tarsal	Calcaneus, Cuboid bone, Intermediate cuneiform bone, Lateral cuneiform bone, Medial cuneiform bone, Navicular bone, Talus bone
Tibia	Lateral condyle of tibia, Medial condyle of tibia, Medial malleolus
Upper Femur	Femoral head, Greater trochanter, Lesser trochanter, Neck of femur

Joints are locations where two or more bones are connected. The acromioclavicular joint in the upper joints body system joins the acromion and clavicle. In the lower joints, the metatarsal-tarsal joint is where the metatarsals and tarsals meet.

Table 2.23.   Upper Joints Body Part key by ICD-10-PCS description

ICD-10-PCS Term	Anatomical Term(s)
Carpal Joint	Intercarpal joint, Midcarpal joint
Cervical Vertebral	Atlantoaxial joint, Cervical facet joint
Cervicothoracic Vertebral	Cervicothoracic facet joint
Elbow Joint	Humeroradial joint, Humeroulnar joint, Proximal radioulnar joint
Finger Phalangeal Joint	Interphalangeal (IP) joint
Metacarpocarpal Joint	Carpometacarpal (CMC) joint
Shoulder Joint	Glenohumeral joint
Thoracic Vertebral Joint	Costotransverse joint, Costovertebral joint, Thoracic facet joint
Thoracolumbar Vertebral Joint	Thoracolumbar facet joint
Wrist Joint	Distal radioulnar joint, Radiocarpal joint

Table 2.24.   Lower Joints Body Part key by ICD-10-PCS description

ICD-10-PCS Term	Anatomical Term(s)
Ankle Joint	Inferior tibiofibular joint, Talocrural joint
Hip Joint	Acetabulofemoral joint
Knee Joint	Femoropatellar joint, Femorotibial joint, Lateral meniscus, Medial meniscus
Lumbar Vertebral Joint	Lumbar facet joint
Lumbosacral Joint	Lumbosacral facet joint
Metatarsal-Phalangeal Joint	Metatarsophalangeal (MTP) joint

Table 2.24.   (Continued)

ICD-10-PCS Term	Anatomical Term(s)
Metatarsal-Tarsal Joint	Tarsometatarsal joint
Sacrococcygeal Joint	Sacrococcygeal symphysis
Tarsal Joint	Calcaneocuboid joint, Cuboideonavicular joint, Cuneonavicular joint, Intercuneiform joint, Subtalar (talocalcaneal) joint, Talocalcaneal (subtalar) joint, Talocalcaneonavicular joint
Toe Phalangeal Joint	Interphalangeal (IP) joint

Urinary System

In ICD-10-PCS, the structures of the urinary system affecting procedural code assignment include the following portions of the urinary system: kidney, kidney pelvis, ureter, bladder, bladder neck, and urethra. Each kidney contains a renal pelvis and two ureters branching from it.

ICD-10-PCS Body Part Key

The ICD-10-PCS terms used to describe a body part may correspond to anatomical terms. To bridge the two, consult table 2.25.

Table 2.25.   Urinary System Body Part key by ICD-10-PCS description

ICD-10-PCS Term	Anatomical Term(s)
Bladder	Trigone of bladder
Kidney	Renal calyx, Renal capsule, Renal cortex, Renal segment
Kidney pelvis	Ureteropelvic junction (UPJ)
Ureter	Ureteral orifice, Ureterovesical orifice
Urethra	Bulbourethral (Cowper's) gland, Cowper's (bulbourethral) gland, External urethral sphincter, Internal urethral sphincter, Membranous urethra, Penile urethra, Prostatic urethra

Female Reproductive System

In ICD-10-PCS, the anatomical portions of the female reproductive system affecting procedural code assignment include the following: ovaries, uterine supporting structures, fallopian tubes, uterus, endometrium, cervix, uterus and cervix, cul-de-sac, vagina, vaginal and Cul-de-sac, clitoris, hymen, vestibular gland, vulva, and ovum.

There are a number of structures that support the uterus. These include pelvic organs, the pelvic diaphragm, along with the broad, round, cardinal, and uterosacral ligaments. The cardinal ligament is also known as the Mackenrodt, lateral cervical ligament, or transverse cervical ligament.

The vulva, the external genitalia of the female, includes the labia majora, mons pubis, labia minora, clitoris, vestibule, vestibule of the vagina, greater and lesser vestibular glands, and vaginal orifice. The greater vestibular glands are also known as Bartholin's glands.

The internal organs include fallopian tubes, ovaries, uterus, and cervix. The uterus consists of the fundus, corpus, cervix, and internal os. The fundus is the top portion (opposite from the cervix), and the corpus is the body. The cervix is the narrow lower portion where the uterus joins to the vagina, and the internal orifice (or internal orifice of cervix uteri or internal os) is the interior narrowing of the uterine cavity. The cul-de-sac is a space behind the uterus and in front of the rectum. Other names for this include the cul-de-sac of Douglas, rectouterine pouch, Douglas' Pouch, or the pouch of Douglas. An ovum or egg cell is produced by the ovaries.

ICD-10-PCS Body Part Key

The ICD-10-PCS terms used to describe a body part may correspond to anatomical terms. To bridge the two, consult table 2.26.

Table 2.26.   Female Reproductive System Body Part key by ICD-10-PCS description

ICD-10-PCS Term	Anatomical Term(s)
Fallopian tube	Oviduct, Salpinx, Uterine tube
Uterine supportive structure	Broad ligament, Infundibulopelvic ligament, Ovarian ligament, Round ligament of uterus

Table 2.26.   (Continued)

ICD-10-PCS Term	Anatomical Term(s)
Uterus	Fundus uteri, Myometrium, Perimetrium, Uterine cornu
Vestibular gland	Bartholin's (greater vestibular) gland, Greater vestibular (Bartholin's) gland, Paraurethral (Skene's) gland, Skene's (paraurethral) gland
Vulva	Labia majora, Labia minora

Male Reproductive System

In ICD-10-PCS, the structures of the male reproductive system affecting procedural code assignment include the following: prostate, seminal vesicle, prostate and seminal vesicles, scrotum, tunica vaginalis, scrotum and tunica vaginalis, testis, spermatic cord, epididymis, epididymis and spermatic cord, vas deferens, penis, prepuce, and male external genitalia.

The overall anatomy of the male reproductive system includes the prostate (gland), seminal vesicle, scrotum, testis, spermatic cord, epididymis, penis, and prepuce (foreskin).

Testicular components are tunica vaginalis, which surrounds a testis to hold it within the scrotum. The spermatic cord suspends it in the scrotum.

ICD-10-PCS Body Part Key

The ICD-10-PCS terms used to describe a body part may correspond to anatomical terms. To bridge the two, consult table 2.27.

Table 2.27.   Male Reproductive System Body Part key by ICD-10-PCS description

ICD-10-PCS Term	Anatomical Term(s)
Penis	Corpus cavernosum, Corpus spongiosum
Prepuce	Foreskin, Glans penis
Vas deferens	Ductus deferens, Ejaculatory duct

Chapter 3

Surgical Approaches

Definitions, Descriptions, and Examples of Surgical Approaches

As mentioned in chapter 1, the fifth character in ICD-10-PCS defines the approach, or the technique used to reach the procedure site. The Medical and Surgical section currently has seven different approach values.

Approaches may be through the skin or mucous membrane, through an orifice, or external.

Approaches through the skin or mucous membranes:

- Open
- Percutaneous
- Percutaneous Endoscopic

Approaches through an orifice:

- Via Natural or Artificial Opening
- Via Natural or Artificial Opening Endoscopic
- Via Natural or Artificial Opening With Percutaneous Endoscopic Assistance

---

The seven approaches and their values are described in table 3.1. The approach comprises three components:

- The access location
- Method
- Type of instrumentation

Table 3.1.   The seven approaches in the Medical and Surgical section

Value	Approach	Definition	Examples
0	Open	Cutting through the skin or mucous membrane and any other body layers necessary to expose the site of the procedure.	Open CABG Open endarterectomy Open resection cecum Abdominal hysterectomy
3	Percutaneous	Entry, by puncture or minor incision, of instrumentation through the skin or mucous membrane and any other body layers necessary to reach the site of the procedure.	Percutaneous needle core biopsy of kidney Liposuction Percutaneous drainage of ascites Needle biopsy of liver
4	Percutaneous Endoscopic	Entry, by puncture or minor incision, of instrumentation through the skin or mucous membrane and any other body layers necessary to reach and visualize the site of the procedure.	Laparoscopic cholecystectomy Laparoscopy with destruction of endometriosis Endoscopic drainage of sinus Arthroscopy
7	Via Natural or Artificial Opening	Entry of instrumentation through a natural or artificial external opening to reach the site of the procedure.	Foley catheter placement Transvaginal intraluminal cervical cerclage Digital rectal exam Endotracheal intubation
8	Via Natural or Artificial Opening Endoscopic	Entry of instrumentation through a natural or artificial external opening to reach and visualize the site of the procedure.	Transurethral cystoscopy with removal bladder stone Endoscopic ERCP Hysteroscopy Colonoscopy EGD Sigmoidoscopy

Table 3.1. (Continued)

Value	Approach	Definition	Examples
F	**Via Natural or Artificial Opening With Percutaneous Endoscopic Assistance**	Entry of instrumentation through a natural or artificial external opening and entry, by puncture or minor incision, of instrumentation through the skin or mucous membrane and any other body layers necessary to aid in the performance of the procedure.	Laparoscopic-assisted vaginal hysterectomy (LAVH)
X	**External**	Procedures performed directly on the skin or mucous membrane and procedures performed indirectly by the application of external force through the skin or mucous membrane.	Resection of tonsils Closed reduction of fracture Excision of skin lesion Cautery nosebleed Manual rupture joint adhesions Reattachment severed ear

ICD-10-PCS Guidelines Applying to Approaches

ICD-10-PCS includes several guidelines pertaining to the correct coding of approaches.

Open Approach with Percutaneous Endoscopic Assistance

B5.2: Procedures performed using the open approach with percutaneous endoscopic assistance are coded to the approach Open.

> **Example:** Laparoscopic-assisted sigmoidectomy is coded to the approach Open.

External Approach

B5.3: Procedures performed within an orifice on structures that are visible without the aid of any instrumentation are coded to the approach External.

> **Example:**   Resection of tonsils is coded to the approach External.

B5.3b: Procedures performed indirectly by the application of external force through the intervening body layers are coded to the approach External.

> **Example:**   Closed reduction of fracture is coded to the approach External.

Percutaneous Procedure via Device

B5.4: Procedures performed percutaneously via a device placed for the procedure are coded to the approach Percutaneous.

> **Example:**   Fragmentation of kidney stone performed via percutaneous nephrostomy is coded to the approach Percutaneous.

The Transition from Coding in ICD-9-CM to ICD-10-PCS

When coding in ICD-9-CM, many procedures do not identify the specific approach as in ICD-10-PCS. In some instances the approach is included in the code title, while other codes do not include any mention of approach.

Examples of ICD-9-CM codes identifying approach:

45.42   Endoscopic polypectomy of large intestine

50.11   Closed (percutaneous) (needle) biopsy of liver

50.12   Open biopsy of liver

50.23   Open ablation of liver lesion or tissue

50.24   Percutaneous ablation of liver lesion or tissue

50.25   Laparoscopic ablation of liver lesion or tissue

53.62   Laparoscopic incisional hernia repair with graft or prosthesis

57.17   Percutaneous cystostomy

Other ICD-9-CM procedures do not specify approach. Some examples are:

29.12   Pharyngeal biopsy
34.23   Biopsy of chest wall
38.50   Ligation and stripping of varicose veins
39.31   Suture of artery
42.91   Ligation of esophageal varices
44.64   Gastropexy
46.71   Suture of laceration of duodenum
52.51   Proximal pancreatectomy
55.4   Partial nephrectomy
58.5   Release urethral stricture
62.5   Orchiopexy
76.11   Biopsy facial bone
80.40   Division of joint capsule, ligament, or cartilage
81.83   Other repair of shoulder
82.41   Suture tendon sheath hand

The important part to learning the approaches is to memorize and apply the definitions and guidelines. For example, the approach called Percutaneous Endoscopic includes a puncture or minor incision, and instrumentation through the skin. This technique describes laparoscopic procedures and arthroscopic procedures. When the scope goes into a natural or artificial opening, such as with colonoscopy or esophagogastroduodenoscopy (EGD), the approach is Via Natural or Artificial Opening Endoscopic.

Careful review of an External approach is indicated. Procedures performed within an orifice on structures that are visible without the aid of any instrumentation would be coded to External. An example is tonsillectomy. Procedures performed indirectly by the application of external force through the intervening body layers are also coded to External. An example is a closed fracture reduction.

Chapter 4

Medical and Surgical Section: Root Operations That Take Out Some/All of a Body Part

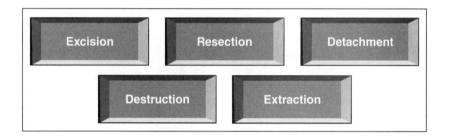

Excision: B

Definition	Cutting out or off, without replacement, a portion of a body part
Explanation	The qualifier Diagnostic is used to identify excision procedures that are biopsies.
Examples	Partial nephrectomy, liver biopsy

Excision is used when a portion of a body part is cut out or off using a sharp instrument. All root operations that employ cutting to accomplish the objective allow the use of any sharp instrument, including but not limited to:

- Scalpel
- Wire
- Scissors
- Bone saw
- Electrocautery tip

Bone Marrow and Endometrial Biopsies: Bone marrow and endometrial biopsies are not coded to Excision. They are coded to Extraction, with the qualifier Diagnostic.

Coding Guideline: B3.4 Biopsy Followed by More Definitive Treatment

If a diagnostic Excision, Extraction, or Drainage procedure (biopsy) is followed by a more definitive procedure, such as Destruction, Excision, or Resection at the same procedure site, both the biopsy and the more definitive treatment are coded.

> **Example:**   Biopsy of breast followed by partial mastectomy at the same procedure site. Both the biopsy and the partial mastectomy procedure are coded.

Coding Guideline: B3.9 Excision for Graft

If an autograft is obtained from a different body part in order to complete the objective of the procedure, a separate procedure is coded.

> **Example:**   Coronary bypass with excision of saphenous vein graft, excision of saphenous vein is coded separately.

Additional Examples of Excision Procedures

- Excision sebaceous cyst right buttock
- Excision malignant melanoma from skin right ear
- Laparoscopy with excision of endometrial implant from left ovary
- Percutaneous needle core biopsy of right kidney
- EGD with gastric biopsy
- Open endarterectomy of left common carotid artery
- Excision of basal cell carcinoma of lower lip
- Open excision of tail of pancreas
- Percutaneous biopsy of right gastrocnemius muscle
- Sigmoidoscopy with sigmoid polypectomy
- Open excision of lesion from right Achilles tendon

Resection: T

Definition   Cutting out or off, without replacement, all of a
                   body part

Explanation N/A

Examples   Total nephrectomy, total lobectomy of lung

Resection is similar to Excision except Resection includes all of a body part, or any subdivision of a body part that has its own body part value in ICD-10-PCS, while Excision includes only a portion of a body part.

Lymph Nodes: When an entire lymph node chain is cut out, the appropriate root operation is Resection. When a lymph node(s) is cut out, the root operation is Excision.

Coding Guideline: B3.8. Excision vs. Resection

PCS contains specific body parts for anatomical subdivisions of a body part, such as lobes of the lungs or liver and regions of the intestine. Resection of the specific body part is coded whenever all of the body part is cut out or off, rather than coding Excision of a less specific body part.

> **Example:** Left upper lung lobectomy is coded to Resection of Upper
> Lung Lobe, Left, rather than Excision of Lung, Left.

The important distinction between excision and resection is if a portion or the entire **body part** is excised. A body part in ICD-10-PCS is not always an entire organ, as some body part values are subdivisions of a particular organ. Body part values may be entire organs, such as the organs of the gallbladder, prostate, or appendix. Some organs—such as the liver, stomach, and lung—have subdivisions of the organ. The liver contains right lobe and left lobe; the stomach includes the pylorus as a specific Body Part; and the lung has multiple body parts (right and left upper lobe, right middle lobe, and right and left lower lobes). Therefore, if the entire right middle lobe of the lung was removed, resection would be assigned rather than excision, because this is a complete body part per ICD-10-PCS. A thorough understanding of the definitions of Excision and Resection root operations is needed, as well as a careful review of the body part values.

When a procedure is performed on the body part, it is necessary to know if the entire body part was excised, but it is also necessary to understand how certain procedures are performed. A prostatectomy is the removal of the prostate; while a transurethral resection of the prostate (TURP) removes the section of the prostate causing symptoms.

It is important to apply the correct root operation regardless of the documentation. It is common to see the terms "removal," "resection," and "excision" used interchangeably. One must identify if the entire body part or part of a body part is excised and apply the ICD-10-PCS body part values correctly.

Additional Examples of Resection Procedures

- Right hemicolectomy
- Open resection of cecum
- Total excision of pituitary gland
- Explantation of left failed kidney
- Open left axillary total lymphadenectomy
- Laparoscopic-assisted total vaginal hysterectomy
- Right total open mastectomy
- Open resection of papillary muscle
- Radical open retropubic prostatectomy
- Laparoscopic cholecystectomy
- Endoscopic bilateral total maxillary sinusectomy

Detachment: 6

Definition	Cutting off all or part of the upper or lower extremities
Explanation	The body part value is the site of the detachment, with a qualifier if applicable to further specify the level where the extremity was detached
Examples	Below knee amputation, disarticulation of shoulder

Detachment represents a narrow range of procedures; it is used exclusively for amputation procedures. Detachment procedure codes are found only in body systems X Anatomical Regions, Upper Extremities and Y Anatomic Regions, Lower Extremities because amputations are performed on extremities, across overlapping body layers, and so could not be coded to a specific musculoskeletal body system such as the bones or joints.

The specific qualifiers used for Detachment are dependent on the body part value in the upper and lower extremities body systems. The definitions in table 4.1 have been developed for qualifiers in both the upper and lower extremities.

Table 4.1. Definitions for qualifiers in the upper and lower extremities

Body Part	Qualifier	Definition
Upper arm and upper leg	1	High: Amputation at the proximal portion of the shaft of the humerus or femur
	2	Mid: Amputation at the middle portion of the shaft of the humerus or femur
	3	Low: Amputation at the distal portion of the shaft of the humerus or femur

Note: The same definitions would be utilized for lower arm and leg.

Table 4.2. Definitions for qualifiers of the hand and foot

Body Part	Qualifier	Definition
Hand and foot	0	Complete
	4	Complete 1st Ray
	5	Complete 2nd Ray
	6	Complete 3rd Ray
	7	Complete 4th Ray
	8	Complete 5th Ray
	9	Partial 1st Ray
	B	Partial 2nd Ray
	C	Partial 3rd Ray
	D	Partial 4th Ray
	F	Partial 5th Ray

When coding amputation of Hand and Foot, these definitions are followed:

Complete: Amputation through the carpometacarpal joint of the hand, or through the tarsal-metatarsal joint of the foot.

Partial: Amputation anywhere along the shaft or head of the metacarpal bone of the hand, or of the metatarsal bone of the foot

Note that the hand and foot are classified using terminology of "ray." These rays refer to the metacarpal and metatarsal bones. The first ray is on the medial side (or the thumb and large toe), then moving to the 5th (or the little finger or toe) on the lateral side.

The metatarsals are the long bones connected to the tarsus (ankle bones). The first ray is connected to the large toe on the medial side (relating to the middle or center), moving to 2nd, 3rd, 4th, and 5th ray on the lateral side.

Table 4.3. Definitions for qualifiers of the thumb, finger, and toe

Body Part	Qualifier	Definition
Thumb, finger, or toe	0	Complete: Amputation at the metacarpophalangeal/metatarsal-phalangeal joint
	1	High: Amputation anywhere along the proximal phalanx
	2	Mid: Amputation through the proximal interphalangeal joint or anywhere along the middle phalanx
	3	Low: Amputation through the distal interphalangeal joint or anywhere along the distal phalanx

Qualifier Value: When a surgeon uses the word "toe" to describe the amputation, but the operative report says he extends the amputation to the midshaft of the 5th metatarsal, which is the foot, the qualifier is Partial 5th Ray.

Additional Examples of Detachment Procedures

- 5th toe ray amputation
- Amputation right elbow level

- 5th ray carpometacarpal joint amputation of left hand
- Right leg and hip amputation through ischium
- DIP joint amputation of right thumb
- Right wrist joint amputation
- Transmetatarsal amputation foot at left big toe
- Midshaft amputation of right humerus
- Left 4th toe amputation at mid-proximal phalanx
- Right above-knee amputation of distal femur

Destruction: 5

Definition	Physical eradication of all or a portion of a body part by the direct use of energy, force, or a destructive agent
Explanation	None of the body part is physically taken out
Examples	Fulguration of rectal polyp, cautery of skin lesion

Destruction "takes out" a body part in the sense that it obliterates the body part so it is no longer there. This root operation defines a broad range of common procedures, because it can be used anywhere in the body to treat a variety of conditions, including:

- Skin and genital warts
- Nasal and colon polyps
- Esophageal varices
- Endometrial implants
- Nerve lesions

Common documentation terms meaning Destruction in ICD-10-PCS are:

- Ablation
- Destruction
- Fulguration
- Cryotherapy
- Cautery
- Coagulation

Additional Examples of Destruction Procedures

- Radiofrequency coagulation of trigeminal nerve
- Cryotherapy of wart on left hand
- Percutaneous radiofrequency ablation of right vocal cord lesion
- Left heart catheterization with laser destruction of arrhythmogenic focus, A-V node
- Cautery of nosebleed
- Cautery of oozing varicose vein of left calf
- Laparoscopy with destruction of endometriosis on both ovaries
- Laser percutaneous coagulation of right retinal vessel hemorrhage
- Talc injection pleurodesis, left side
- Sclerotherapy of brachial plexus lesion with alcohol injection
- Fulguration of endometrium

Extraction: D

Definition	Pulling or stripping out or off all or a portion of a body part by the use of force
Explanation	The qualifier Diagnostic is used to identify extraction procedures that are biopsies
Examples	Dilation and curettage, vein stripping leg

Extraction is coded when the method employed to take out the body part is pulling or stripping. Minor cutting, such as that used in vein stripping procedures, is included in Extraction if the objective of the procedure is nevertheless met by pulling or stripping. As with all applicable ICD-10-PCS codes, cutting used to reach the procedure site is specified in the approach value.

To help understand the intent of Extraction, gaining knowledge about how the procedures are performed in the two examples may be helpful. In the curettage (meaning scraping), a sharp instrument is used to scrape or suction away the lining of the uterus. The Dilation is not additionally coded because the dilation would be considered a component of the procedure necessary to complete the objective or, in other words, the dilation must be done in order to complete the curettage.

This would be necessary to reach the procedure site, and is only being performed to accomplish the curettage.

In the vein stripping, two small incisions are made in the leg, near the top and bottom of the damaged vein. The surgeon threads a thin flexible plastic wire through the vein toward the other cut. As the wire is pulled out through the lower cut, the head of the wire pulls the vein down and out. This procedure may also be done using hooks.

Once again, be careful of documentation. It is important to convert common terminology to the appropriate root operation according to the intent of the procedure. For example, the procedure documentation may say removal, but in actuality, using PCS definitions, an extraction was performed. Removal of a thumbnail would be coded to Extraction. The root operation of Removal is not correct because by definition a Removal in ICD-10-PCS is defined as taking out or off a device from a body part.

Additional Examples of Extraction Procedures

- Extraction of teeth
- Suction dilation & curettage
- Removal left thumbnail
- Phacoemulsification cataract without replacement
  - A phacoemulsification with IOL implant is classified to the root operation Replacement. Remember that this group of root operations includes taking out, but not replacement.
- Laparoscopy with needle aspiration of ova for in-vitro fertilization
- Non-excisional debridement of skin ulcer, right foot
  - An excisional debridement is classified to the root operation Excision.
- Open stripping of abdominal fascia, right side
- Hysteroscopy with D&C
- Liposuction for medical purposes, left upper arm
  - A liposuction for cosmetic reasons is coded to the root operation Alteration.
- Removal of tattered right ear drum fragments with tweezers
- Microincisional phlebectomy of spider veins, right lower leg
- Bone marrow biopsy
- Endometrial biopsy (See note in Excision section)

Apply Knowledge to Transition from Coding in ICD-9-CM to ICD-10-PCS

Case Example #1

The following case is for an EGD with biopsy of the duodenum, which is coded to 45.16 in ICD-9-CM. The code descriptor for 45.16 is Esophagogastroduodenoscopy (EGD) with closed biopsy and is categorized under category 45.1, Diagnostic procedures on small intestine.

Case Description: A 65-year-old patient had experienced blood in his stools (melena) for the past several days. During the past 12 hours, the bleeding increased, and the patient felt very weak and dizzy. He was admitted to the hospital by his physician and advised to have an upper GI endoscopy (EGD), to which he agreed. The EGD was performed, and the patient was found to have an area of erosion, ulceration, and bleeding as seen in the duodenum during the EGD examination. A biopsy of the duodenum was taken during the EGD. The physician's diagnosis was acute duodenal ulceration with hemorrhage.

Case Explanation: A biopsy in ICD-10-PCS is classified to Drainage or Excision, depending on the intent of the procedure. In this case, the biopsy was documented to have been taken at the duodenum, with no mention of drainage. The case would code to the root operation Excision (0DB98ZX) in ICD-10-PCS. Note that in ICD-10-PCS the specific body part (duodenum) can be identified by the body part value of 9. In the Excision root operation, diagnostic procedures (biopsies) are identified by the value of "X" in the seventh character. Coding Guideline B3.11a states that inspection of a body part performed in order to achieve the objective of a procedure is not coded separately. Therefore, the Inspection (EGD) is not coded.

Case Example #2

The following case is for a right breast lumpectomy for carcinoma, which is coded to 85.21 in ICD-9-CM. The code descriptor for 85.21 is Local excision of lesion of breast and is categorized under category 85.2, Excision or destruction of breast tissue.

Case Description:

History: A 55-year-old woman presented to the office with a right breast mass, approximately 2.0 cm × 2.0 cm, in the upper inner quadrant.

There was no lymphadenopathy. She has a significant family history of breast cancer being diagnosed in her mother, maternal aunt, and older sister. Three days ago, a fine needle aspiration procedure demonstrated cells suspicious for malignancy. She was admitted to the hospital for definitive surgical treatment with a right breast lumpectomy.

Operative Findings: A hard 2.0 × 2.0 cm mass in the upper inner quadrant of the right breast with no lymphadenopathy was confirmed. Pathology reports the specimen to be confirmed as carcinoma. The surgical margins on the mass excised were found to be normal.

Procedure: After preoperative counseling, the patient was taken to the operating room and placed in a supine position on the table. The chest, right breast, and shoulder were prepped with Betadine scrub and paint and draped in the usual sterile fashion. The skin around the mass was anesthetized with 1% lidocaine solution. An elliptical incision was made, leaving a 1.5 cm margin around the mass in a circumferential fashion. The mass was sharply excised down to the pectoralis fascia, which was excised and sent with the specimen of the breast. The deep medial aspect of the specimen was marked with a long suture and the deep inferior margin marked with a short suture. The wound was left open until the pathologist returned the call that the margins were negative under frozen section. The wound was copiously irrigated. Hemostasis was achieved with Bovie cauterization and 3-0 Vicryl suture ligatures. The skin was closed with a running subcuticular 4-0 Vicryl, Benzoin and steri-strips. A sterile dressing was applied. The patient was subsequently transferred to the recovery room in stable condition. She tolerated the procedure well and will be advised of the procedural findings when she is returned to her room.

Case Explanation: The lumpectomy would code to the root operation Excision (0H**B**T0ZZ) in ICD-10-PCS. The lumpectomy involves removing the lesion and enough surrounding tissue to establish clear margins, but the entire breast is not removed. The simple mastectomy, which resects the entire breast, is very different from a lumpectomy. The mastectomy would be coded to the root operation Resection.

The procedure includes documentation that this was done in an open technique so the approach for the fifth character is 0. The procedure was a therapeutic procedure, and not diagnostic, so even though the tissue was sent to pathology, the qualifier of Z is used, not X for diagnostic.

Case Example #3

The following case is for a debridement of the patella, which is coded to 77.66 in ICD-9-CM. The code descriptor for 77.66 is Local excision of lesion or tissue of patella and is categorized under category 77.6, Local excision of lesion or tissue of bone.

Case Description:

History: This is a 65-year-old man who is currently in the hospital under the care of his internal medicine physician for treatment of a duodenal ulcer, GERD, and an enlarged prostate with urinary retention. He has been seen by an urologist and has had a cystoscopic examination. He is medically under control at this time and will be ready for discharge in a day or so. He was referred to orthopedics for the complaint of severe left knee pain that is limiting his mobility. He states he has had no particular trauma to the knee but has always felt the left knee to be his "bad knee." The patient wants a knee replacement because his 75-year-old brother had one in the past 6 months and is back to golfing twice a week. This patient cannot walk the nine holes on the golf course as he was able to do last year. X-ray examination of the left knee is not striking, with some arthritic changes noted but no major pathology suspected. The patient consented to an arthroscopic examination of the knee to determine what treatment can be recommended.

Operative Findings: An arthroscopic debridement of the left patella was performed. The medical meniscus, lateral meniscus, and ACL were completely normal. Examination of the patellofemoral joints allowed appreciation of the magnitude of the problem with the patella. The entire surface of the patella was involved with chondromalacia with surfaces graded from 3 to mostly 4. He also has a significant degree of prepatellar bursitis of the left knee that likely is also contributing to his pain and stiffness. The pros and cons of a left knee arthroplasty will be discussed with the patient after he recovers from this procedure and determination of pain relief after this debridement is assessed.

Procedure: The patient was provided general endotracheal tube anesthesia, and the left lower extremity was prepared and draped in the usual manner for arthroscopic surgery of the left knee. After insufflation of lidocaine and epinephrine, three standard portals, two medial and one lateral, were established in the usual manner. There was difficulty in evaluating the suprapatellar pouch as well as the patellofemoral joint

initially because of the extensive chondromalacia and synovial reac-
tion. Prepatellar bursitis was also present. The medial compartment was
first able to be evaluated carefully, and the medial meniscus was found
to be completely normal to observation and to probing, as were the
medial femoral condyle and medial tibial plateau. The ACL appeared
to be intact. The lateral meniscus and lateral compartment were, in
general, completely normal. In order to see the contents of the femoral-
tibial joint, some debridement of pedunculated synovial tissue was
necessary. On returning to the patellofemoral joint, some debridement
was done. At this point, the magnitude of the problem on the patella
was evident. Essentially the entire surface of the patella was involved
with chondromalacia. There was mostly grade-4 chondromalacia over
more of the lateral facet but also on the medial facet with grade-3 chondromalacia. This involved a large portion of the main articular surface
of the patella. At the conclusion of this procedure, instrumentation was
removed and sterile dressings applied. The patient was awakened and
taken to the recovery room in stable condition.

Case Explanation: The debridement of the patella would code to the
root operation Excision (0Q**B**F4ZZ) in ICD-10-PCS. Excision is used
because the entire patella was not removed. The procedure was performed laparoscopically so the approach is percutaneous endoscopic (4).
The patella, also known as the knee cap, is a thick, circular-triangular
bone which articulates with the femur and covers and protects the anterior articular surface of the knee joint. Overuse, injury, or other condition may lead to chondromalacia of the patella (CMP), or damage to the
cartilage under the patella.

Case Example #4

In this case, code only the discectomy.

The following case is for a discectomy of the disk herniation at L5-S1,
which is coded to 80.51 in ICD-9-CM. The code descriptor for 80.51 is
Excision of intervertebral disc and is categorized under category 80.5,
Excision, destruction and other repair of intervertebral disc.

Case Description:

History: The patient is a 38-year-old male with a 2-month history of
lower back pain radiating down the left leg. The patient reported that

he had suffered a work-related injury while acting as a commercial driver and while assisting in the cleanup of the New Orleans hurricane Katrina disaster. Because of the severe pain, he was unable to work so he returned home. An MRI of the lumbar spine taken 2 weeks ago shows a large extruded disk herniation on the left side, L5-S1, causing severe nerve impingement. He has failed conservative treatment and is now indicated for nerve root decompression. He reports weakness in the left leg but denies any problems with bowel or bladder control. There is moderate tension in the lower back with flexion to 70 degrees and extension to 10 degrees secondary to lower back pain. He also complains of intermittent pain and numbness in his right hand and fingers that was evaluated during this preoperative episode, and he was diagnosed with right carpal tunnel syndrome. We will consider surgically correcting the carpal tunnel problem after he recovers from this procedure. His past surgical history is a left knee arthroscopy 12 years ago. He has no medical problems other than his back and the carpal tunnel syndrome in his right upper extremity. His preoperative diagnosis is acute left L5-S1 radiculopathy secondary to large L5-S1 disk herniation. He was admitted to the hospital for surgery.

Operative Findings: The patient had a L5-S1 laminectomy and discectomy. The nerve root was resting freely at the conclusion of the procedures, and there was no dural injury.

Procedure: After satisfactory induction of general anesthesia, AV boots were applied to both feet. The patient was turned to the prone position on a Kambin frame. Care was taken to make sure that pressure points were well padded. Once the position of the back was judged to be satisfactory, it was prepped and draped in the usual fashion. Epinephrine 1:500,000 solution was injected into the planned surgical incision site in the right lower back. Sharp dissection was carried down to the level of the fascia. The fascia was incised and subperiosteal dissection was carried out along the spinous processes down to the lamina and facet of each vertebral level. Deep retractors were then used to place a marker and intraoperative fluoroscopy confirmed the L5-S1 level. Once oriented to our level, the laminotomy was begun. The ligamentum flavum was debrided. A partial facetectomy of approximately 10% was carried out on the left side. This allowed identification of the nerve root. Upon retracting the nerve root we could immediately identify extruded disc fragment. We were able to retrieve a moderate-sized fragment.

Further inspection up behind the body of L5 produced a large extruded fragment. Exploration of the annular defect area identified only a tiny amount of loose material, all of which was retrieved. After multiple inspections, we were satisfied that all of the loose fragments of the disc had been removed. The nerve root was resting freely. Satisfactory hemostasis was achieved. There was no dural injury. A dry piece of Gelfoam was placed over the laminotomy defects. The fascial layer was closed with #1 Vicryl. The subcutaneous layer was closed with 2-0 Vicryl, and the skin was closed with 4-0 Monocryl. The patient was turned to the supine position on the hospital bed and awakened in the operating room. The patient was noted to have intact bilateral lower extremity motor function when asked to move both of his legs, which he could do. The patient was extubated in the operating room and taken to recovery in good condition.

Case Explanation: This discectomy would code to the root operation Excision (0SB40ZZ) in ICD-10-PCS. In ICD-9-CM, the procedure assigned is excision. In ICD-10-PCS however, choices are available for resection or excision. To select the root operation code, the intent of the procedure must be known. The documentation above discusses removing fragments of the disc, so in this case excision was selected. If documentation substantiates that the entire disc was removed, then resection would be selected. Under discectomy in the Index, the body system is provided as either upper or lower joints. The L5-S1 is lower joint because it is below the diaphragm. Lumbosacral disc (4) is a body part in the Lower Joint body system. The laminectomy is not coded separately because it is a procedural step necessary to reach the operative site (B3.1b).

A herniated disk is a protrusion of the nucleus pulposus or annulus fibrosus of the intervertebral disk, which may impinge on nerve roots.

Case Example #5

In this case, do not code the nuclear medicine bone scan.

The following case is for an endoscopic diagnostic biopsy of the right main bronchus, which is coded to 33.24 in ICD-9-CM. The code descriptor for 33.24 is Closed (endoscopic) biopsy of bronchus and is categorized under category 33.2, Diagnostic procedures on lung and bronchus.

Case Description: A 75-year-old male patient, known to have emphysema, was advised by his physician to be admitted to the hospital to evaluate and treat his worsening lung condition. The patient complained that his coughing and wheezing had become worse and his sputum was streaked with blood. A chest x-ray done on an outpatient basis the previous week showed a mass in the main bronchus. A fiberoptic bronchoscopy and needle biopsy of the bronchial mass was performed. The pathologic diagnosis of the biopsy examination was small cell type bronchogenic carcinoma located in the right main bronchus. A nuclear medicine bone scan found areas of suspicious lesions that were determined to be bone metastasis. The diagnoses provided by the physician at discharge were bronchogenic, small cell carcinoma of the right main bronchus with metastatic disease in the bones and emphysema.

Case Explanation: The bronchoscopy with the needle biopsy of the right main bronchus would code to the root operation Excision (0B**B**38ZX) in ICD-10-PCS. The body part for the fourth character is main bronchus, right (3) and the approach is via natural or artificial opening endoscopic because it was performed during the bronchoscopy (fifth character 8). The seventh character qualifier of X is used to show that the biopsy was done for diagnostic purposes. During a bronchoscopy the scope (either rigid or flexible) is inserted and advanced down the trachea into the bronchial system.

Case Example #6

The following case is for the excision of a malignant skin lesion, which is coded to 86.3 in ICD-9-CM. The code descriptor for 86.3 is Other local excision or destruction of lesion or tissue of skin and subcutaneous tissue and is categorized under category 86, Operations on skin and subcutaneous tissue. Of note is that in ICD-9-CM all sites code to the same code except for some isolated sites (breast, nose, and scrotum). Further, skin and subcutaneous tissue are assigned to the same code.

Case Description: This is a 65-year-old woman who has biopsy-proven malignant melanoma of the right calf. The pathology diagnosis was superficial spreading of malignant melanoma. The patient is brought to the hospital outpatient department for excision of the 2.5 × 1.5 cm skin lesion. She will be seen in the office for suture removal and a discussion on what further treatment might be indicated.

Case Explanation: The excision of a skin lesion would code to the root operation Excision (0H**B**KXZZ) in ICD-10-PCS. Skin (rather than subcutaneous tissue) was selected because of the documentation that this was a lesion of the skin and that it was superficial. But when an operative report is available, careful review of the report is indicated to see actually how deep the excision went. Note that when excisions are performed on the skin, the approach is external. This procedure was therapeutic and not diagnostic because the biopsy was done previously. It is important to know when coding if the procedure is being done on the skin or the subcutaneous layers.

Case Example #7

The following case is for a closed biopsy of the brain (parietal lobe), which is coded to 01.13 in ICD-9-CM. The code descriptor for 01.13 is Closed (percutaneous) (needle) biopsy of brain and is categorized under category 01.1, Diagnostic procedures on skull, brain, and cerebral meninges. Code 01.13 includes burr hole approach and/or stereotactic method.

Case Description: The patient is a 52-year-old painter who was washing windows at his home with his wife one day prior to admission when he developed what he called the "mother of all headaches" or the worst headache of his life. He had nausea but no vomiting. He later noticed visual disturbances and dizziness. Thinking the headache would go away; he went to bed but was unable to sleep all night because of the intensity of the headache pain, which was not relieved by Tylenol. He called his physician the next morning and was advised to go to the Emergency Department, where he was admitted. CT and MRI scans of the head and chest were abnormal. The MRI of the head found a three ring-enhancing lesion located in the parietal area associated with a large amount of edema extending into the occipital and temporal regions. The CT of the chest found pulmonary lesions that seem to be cavitating in the right lower lobe. The patient had smoked for the past 40 years. The patient consented to and had performed the following procedure: closed biopsy of the brain through a burr hole approach. Based on the pathological findings, the physician concluded the patient had a glioblastoma multiforme of the parietal region. In addition to these diagnoses, the physician gave other final diagnoses of pre-diabetes and smoker. The patient was discharged home as he wished to seek a second opinion at a major university medical center. Copies of his records and radiology films were given to the patient for this purpose. The CT of the lung will be addressed when treatment for the GBM is determined.

Case Explanation: A brain biopsy of the parietal lobe of the brain would code to the root operation Excision (00**B**73ZX) in ICD-10-PCS. The parietal lobe is part of the cerebrum and ICD-10-PCS classifies it to Cerebral Hemisphere. (Page A.18 of Appendix A [ICD-10-PCS definitions] of the ICD-10-PCS Reference Manual).

The burr is a type of surgical drill used for making holes in bone (Dorland 2003). Because entry is better described as puncture than cutting through skin or mucous membrane to expose the site of the procedure, percutaneous is selected as the approach. The seventh character (X) identifies the biopsy procedure.

The parietal lobe is a lobe in the brain positioned superior to the occipital lobe and posterior to the frontal lobe.

Case Example #8

The following case is for an excisional debridement of skin ulcers. The debridement of the buttock ulcer is coded to 83.45 in ICD-9-CM. The code descriptor for 83.45 is Other myectomy and is categorized under category 83.4, Other excision of muscle, tendon, and fascia. The debridement of the heel skin ulcer is coded to 86.22 in ICD-9-CM. The code descriptor for 86.22 is Excisional debridement of wound, infection, or burn and is categorized under category 86.2, Excision or destruction of lesion or tissue of skin and subcutaneous tissue.

Case Description: A 90-year-old woman, a resident of a long-term care facility, was admitted to the hospital with a severe decubitus ulcer on the right buttock described as a stage 4 pressure ulcer. The patient also had a small chronic ulcer on the right heel. The patient also has generalized atherosclerosis. Treatments of the skin conditions were an excisional debridement of the skin of the heel and an open excisional debridement into the muscle of the buttock (superficial gluteus maximus of trunk). The wound care nurse closely monitored the patient after surgery and gave detailed instructions to the nurses at the long-term care facility who would be taking care of the patient after discharge. The patient was transferred back to the long-term care facility. The wound care physician and nurse would visit the patient in the long-term care facility within 1 week to monitor the healing of the pressure and chronic ulcers.

Case Explanation: The excisional debridement into the muscle would code to the root operation Excision (0K**B**F0ZZ) in ICD-10-PCS. The gluteus maximus is the largest and most superficial muscle of the buttock. It is interesting in the ICD-10-PCS Definitions list (In Appendix A of the 2010 ICD-10-PCS Reference Manual, gluteus maximus muscle is listed with Muscle, Trunk (page A.26) and with Muscle, Hip (page A.24). This may be because the muscle is a large muscle, and the location of the procedure may be more in line with the trunk, or more to the side in the hip area.

The excisional debridement of the skin of the right heel would code to the root operation Excision (0H**B**MXZZ) in ICD-10-PCS. There is no body part for heel in ICD-10-PCS so foot is used. The approach is external. It would be correct to code this second procedure because of coding guideline B3.2.a. stating that multiple procedures are performed if the same root operation is performed on different body parts as defined by distinct values of the body part character.

Case Example #9

The following case is for a skin biopsy, which is coded to 86.11 in ICD-9-CM. The code descriptor for 86.11 is Biopsy of skin and subcutaneous tissue and is categorized under category 86.1, Diagnostic procedures on skin and subcutaneous tissue.

Case Description: A 60-year-old man was sent to the dermatologist's office by his primary care physician for evaluation of several lesions on his arms and legs. The patient states he spends a lot of time out of doors as a mailman and golfing every weekend. The patient expresses the concern that he may have skin cancer. He remembers that his father, a farmer, had many of these same types of lesions on his arms and neck through the years. After performing a thorough skin examination, the physician finds multiple brown annular keratotic lesions on the patient's arms and lower legs with patchy dry areas around them.

The physician performs a shave skin biopsy of the patient's right upper arm and examines the lesion microscopically. No cancer type cells are seen. Given the patient's history of the same lesions in the family and his frequent exposure to ultraviolet sunlight, the physician explains to the patient that he has what is referred to as DSAP or disseminated superficial actinic porokeratosis. Further he explains there is no treatment to prevent these lesions from returning once removed. The patient elects not to have any lesions removed at this time but will consider it and make an appointment in the future if he decides to have them removed.

Case Explanation: The shave skin biopsy procedure would code to the root operation Excision (0H**B**BXZX) in ICD-10-PCS. Even though the patient had multiple lesions, only the right upper arm was biopsied.

Case Example #10

The following case is for an arthroscopic partial medial meniscectomy of his right knee, which is coded to 80.6 in ICD-9-CM. The code descriptor for 80.6 is Excision of semilunar cartilage of knee and is categorized under category 80, Incision and excision of joint structures.

Case Description: The patient is a 56-year-old man with significant hypertensive heart disease who was admitted to the hospital for an arthroscopic partial medial meniscectomy on his right knee. Given his hypertension and heart disease, the cardiologist advised the orthopedic surgeon to admit the patient to the hospital for at least overnight monitoring after the procedure. During a previous orthopedic surgery, this patient had a hypertensive crisis and was placed in the intensive care unit for monitoring. This surgery was performed uneventfully. The patient had an arthroscopic partial medial meniscectomy of the posterior horn of the medical meniscus. This was determined to be an old tear, likely from a football playing injury. There were no loose bodies in the medial and lateral gutters. The articular cartilage surfaces were in reasonably good condition. The notches of the anterior cruciate and posterior cruciate ligaments were intact. Within the lateral compartment, the meniscus was intact and the articular cartilage surfaces in good condition. At the conclusion of the procedure, all excess fluid was drained, the portal incisions closed with nylon sutures, an injection of Marcaine was administered for pain control, and sterile dressings were

applied. The patient was taken to the recovery room and then transferred to a regular bed. He was discharged the following morning with
a follow up-appointment with the surgeon in 10 days.

Case Explanation: The partial meniscectomy would code to the
root operation Excision (0SBC4ZZ) in ICD-10-PCS. The body system is Lower Joints (S), and the body part is Knee Joint, Right (C).
The approach is percutaneous endoscopic because it was performed
arthroscopically.

Case Example #11

The following case is for a total open abdominal hysterectomy and
bilateral salpingo-oophorectomy. The hysterectomy is coded to 68.49
in ICD-9-CM. The code descriptor for 68.49 is Other and unspecified
total abdominal hysterectomy and is categorized under category 68.4,
Total abdominal hysterectomy. The BSO is coded to 65.61 in ICD-
9-CM. The code descriptor for 65.61 is Other removal of both ovaries
and tubes at same operative episode and is categorized under category
65.6, Bilateral salpingo-oophorectomy.

Case Description: A 59-year-old woman was admitted to the hospital
for a scheduled open total abdominal hysterectomy (TAH) with a bilateral salpingo-oophorectomy (BSO). The patient also had type 2 diabetes which was well-controlled by medications. The patient first visited
her gynecologist several months ago complaining of postmenopausal
vaginal bleeding and abnormal vaginal discharge. An endometrial
biopsy was taken in the office and was suggestive of uterine cancer. The
TAH-BSO was performed, and the following postoperative diagnoses
were recorded by the physician: Stage I endometrial adenocarcinoma
(corpus uteri) and bilateral corpus luteum cysts of the ovaries, worse
on the right side. The patient continued to receive oral diabetic medications while in the hospital.

Case Explanation: TAH and BSO would code to the root operation
Resection (0UT90ZZ, 0UTC0ZZ, 0UT20ZZ and 0UT70ZZ) in ICD-10-
PCS. Resection is selected because the complete Body Part is removed.
Four codes are required for this procedure. A total hysterectomy
includes resection or removal of both the uterus and cervix. Note that
all four codes have the very same composition except for the fourth

character (body part). All codes can be obtained from the same ICD-10-PCS table, with correct selection of the body parts. The uterus is body part 9, the cervix is C, the bilateral ovaries are 2, and the bilateral fallopian tubes are 7.

Case Example #12

The following case is for a laparoscopic cholecystectomy, which is coded to 51.23 in ICD-9-CM. The code descriptor for 51.23 is Laparoscopic cholecystectomy and is categorized under category 51.2, Cholecystectomy. Also, the laparoscopic biopsy of the liver would be coded to 50.14 in ICD-9-CM. The code descriptor for 50.14 is Laparoscopic liver biopsy and is categorized under category 50.1, Diagnostic procedures on liver.

Case Description:

History: This is a 72-year-old man who presented with a history of epigastric pain for several months. This lasts 3–4 hours each time, and has been occurring every 2–3 days. He has been nauseated, although there was no vomiting. He has had the urge to go to the bathroom for frequent bowel movements after meals. He has tried to avoid greasy food and has been placed on Nexium, but this only helped to some extent. An ultrasound was performed on the gallbladder, and gallstones were found. An upper GI x-ray showed mild esophageal motility problems with a hiatal hernia. He gets a screening PSA every year and has had a colonoscopy, which was normal. He consented to a laparoscopic cholecystectomy and was admitted to the hospital.

Operative Findings: The laparoscopic examination revealed evidence of inflammation of a chronic nature of the gallbladder along with gallstones. There was also a nodule on the liver on the inferior surface on the right lateral aspect of the gallbladder fossa. The rest of the visualized viscera were unremarkable. After pathologic examination, the postoperative diagnoses are cholelithiasis with chronic cholecystitis with a bile duct adenoma.

Procedure: The patient was prepared and draped in the usual fashion. An umbilical incision was made. A Veress needle was introduced with a sheath and pneumoperitoneum was established with the usual precautions. Then an 11-mm port was placed. A laparoscope was introduced.

Under direct vision an operative port in the right upper quadrant and two 5-mm lateral ports were placed. A laparoscopic examination revealed evidence of inflammation of a chronic nature of the gallbladder with gallstones. There was also a nodule in the liver. The rest of the viscera visualized were normal. The cholecystectomy was done by gently grasping the fundus. The neck was then grasped. The Calot's Triangle was then exposed. The anatomy was carefully defined. The cystic duct and the cystic artery were traced up to the neck of the gallbladder. Herein it was secured with hemoclips, divided, and closed to the neck of the gallbladder. Then it was completely dissected off of the gallbladder bed and retrieved in an Endopouch and removed. Irrigation was carried out. Excellent hemostasis was ascertained. Following this, an evaluation of the nodule was carried out using a hook cautery. The surrounding borders of this nodule, in the right inferior surface of the lobe of the liver, were cauterized. Then a small wedge biopsy of this tissue was taken. The base was cauterized. This tissue was then sent, with the gallbladder tissue, for histopathological analysis. At this point, having ascertained good hemostasis, all the ports were removed under direct vision. The fascia was closed with 0 Vicryl sutures. Subcutaneous tissue was closed with 0 Vicryl sutures. The skin was closed with 4-0 Monocryl. Marcaine 0.5% with epinephrine was injected to achieve postoperative analgesia. The patient tolerated the procedure well and was stable at the end of the procedure and taken to recovery.

Case Explanation: The laparoscopic cholecystectomy would code to the root operation Resection (0F**T**44ZZ) in ICD-10-PCS. The entire gallbladder was removed so this is resection. There was also a biopsy done of the right lobe of the liver. This would code to the root operation Excision (0F**B**14ZX) in ICD-10-PCS. A biopsy is excision rather than resection, and the seventh character identifies the biopsy with the X.

Case Example #13

The following case is for a laparoscopic appendectomy, which is coded to 47.01 in ICD-9-CM. The code descriptor for 47.01 is Laparoscopic appendectomy and is categorized under category 47.0, Appendectomy.

Case Description: A 64-year-old man was seen in his physician's office with a variety of gastrointestinal complaints, including vague, abdominal pain, diarrhea, urinary frequency, and flushing across his face, neck and chest. Laboratory and radiology tests were inconclusive, but based on his continuing symptoms; the physician suspected the patient might have a chronic form of appendicitis. An outpatient laparoscopic complete appendectomy was performed in the hospital ambulatory surgery department. A frozen section was requested during the procedure and the findings returned were "suspected carcinoid tumor of the appendix awaiting final histopathological exam." Upon recovery from the anesthesia, the patient agreed to be admitted the same day. Further pathology studies confirmed the diagnosis of malignant carcinoid tumor of the appendix. Other testing found that the patient was experiencing a "carcinoid syndrome" because of this tumor, which explained many of his vague symptoms, including the flushing. The appendectomy is considered curative treatment for the appendiceal tumor. Upon discharge, the patient will be seen in the oncologist office for further recommendations, especially to treat the carcinoid syndrome.

Case Explanation: The laparoscopic appendectomy would code to the root operation Resection (0DTJ4ZZ) in ICD-10-PCS. There is no evidence that only a portion of the appendix was removed, in fact the documentation states "complete" appendectomy. It would be necessary to review medical record documentation carefully to make this determination. Even though a diagnosis was made, this would not be considered a diagnostic biopsy because the entire appendix was removed.

Case Example #14

The following case is for a therapeutic splenectomy, which is coded to 41.5 in ICD-9-CM. The code descriptor for 41.5 is Total splenectomy and is categorized under category 41, Operations on bone marrow and spleen.

Case Description: The patient, a 40-year-old man, was diagnosed with acquired hemolytic anemia, autoimmune type with warm-reactive (IgG) antibodies, and had been treated with glucocorticoids (prednisone.) The patient failed to respond to this medication. The patient is also under treatment for systemic lupus erythematosus. Given the aggressive nature of his anemia, he was advised to be admitted to the hospital and have a splenectomy to eliminate the body's further destruction of red blood cells. The open splenectomy was performed without complications, and the patient was discharged to be followed in the physician and surgeon's offices.

Case Explanation: The splenectomy would code to the root operation Resection (07**T**P0ZZ) in ICD-10-PCS. The spleen is part of the Lymphatic and hemic systems (7). Documentation indicates that this procedure was performed in an open approach.

Case Example #15

The following case is for a bilateral tonsillectomy, which is coded to 28.2 in ICD-9-CM. The code descriptor for 28.2 is Tonsillectomy without adenoidectomy and is categorized under category 28, Operations on tonsils and adenoids.

Case Description: A bilateral tonsillectomy was performed on a 9-year-old patient to resolve his recurring infections due to tonsillar hyperplasia. No infection is present at the time of the surgery. The patient was admitted as an inpatient for an overnight stay.

Case Explanation: The bilateral tonsillectomy would code to the root operation Resection (0C**T**PXZZ) in ICD-10-PCS. There is no evidence that the tonsils were not resected in total. In fact, the procedure was a bilateral procedure. The documentation is not very specific regarding the approach. It was elected to assign External because of Coding Guideline B5.3.a—Procedures performed within an orifice on structures that are visible without the aid of any instrumentation are coded to the approach External. The surgical operative report would be reviewed to substantiate this information.

Case Example #16

The following case is for an amputation of the toe. The amputation was extended to the midshaft of the 5th metatarsal and this is coded to 84.12 in ICD-9-CM. The code descriptor for 84.12 is Amputation through foot and is categorized under category 84.1, Amputation of lower limb. Code 84.12 includes transmetatarsal amputation.

Case Description: This 65-year-old patient is having an amputation of the left toe because of severe osteomyelitis. The procedure was performed in the following manner. A semi-elliptical incision was made around the base of the left toe with a #15 blade without difficulty. Careful sharp dissection was made down to the bone, and care was taken to avoid the 4th toe's neurovascular bundle. There was obvious osteomyelitis of the proximal phalanx of the fifth toe and the toe itself was disarticulated, the proximal head of the fifth lower extremity meta-tarsal, without difficulty. Specimens were sent to pathology for culture and examination.

Next, both sharp and blunt dissection were used to adequately expose the head of the fifth metatarsal, and this was done without dif-ficulty. A small rongeur was then used to remove the head of the fifth metatarsal, and soft spongy bone was felt beneath this area. Examina-tion of the patient's x-rays revealed that there was an area of cortical lucency at the base of the head of the fifth metatarsal, and the decision was made to extend the amputation to the midshaft of the fifth meta-tarsal, and the transmetatarsal amputation was done without difficulty using a rongeur. The wound was then flushed with normal saline, and bleeding viable tissue was observed throughout the wound. There was adequate flap coverage of the remaining fifth metatarsal.

Case Explanation: The amputation procedure would code to the root operation Detachment (0Y**6**N0ZF) in ICD-10-PCS. The surgeon uses the word toe to describe the amputation, but the operative report says that it was extends to the midshaft of the fifth metatarsal and was a transmetatarsal amputation. This qualifies as the body part of foot (N) and the qualifier would be partial 5th ray.

Case Example #17

The following case is for a conization of the cervix by cryotherapy, which is coded to 67.33 in ICD-9-CM. The code descriptor for 67.33 is Destruction of lesion of cervix by cryosurgery and is categorized under category 67.3, Other excision or destruction of lesion or tissue of cervix.

Case Description: A 40-year-old woman with known moderate cervi-cal dysplasia had been seen in the outpatient surgery department the previous week for a colposcopy and biopsy. Today the patient returns for a conization of the cervix by cryosurgery. The vaginal canal was opened with the speculum and the cervix visualized. The cryo probe was inserted and placed on the surface of the abnormal tissue on the cervix. There were no complications. The patient will follow-up in the office.

Case Explanation: The cryosurgery of the cervix would code to the root operation Destruction (0U**5**C7ZZ) in ICD-10-PCS. The fifth char-acter approach would be via natural or artificial opening (7).

Case Example #18

The following case is for a fulguration of the ureter, which is coded to 56.41. The code descriptor for 56.41 is Partial ureterotomy and is categorized under category 56.4, Ureterectomy. There is no code for the site of ureter under destruction, fulguration, or electrocoagulation in ICD-9-CM, so the code is not as specific as it can be in ICD-10-PCS.

Case Description:

Operative Report

Preoperative Diagnosis: Recurrent right ureteral malignancy

Postoperative Diagnosis: Same

Procedure: Under satisfactory standby anesthesia, the patient was placed in the dorsolithotomy position. Her external genitalia were prepped and draped in sterile fashion for a cystourethroscopy examination.

Two percent Xylocaine jelly was instilled into the urethra for topical anesthesia. Using a #20 Wappler panendoscope sheath, right angle, and four oblique fiberoptic telescopes, a cystourethroscopy was performed with a normal urethra noted. The bladder was also unremarkable but showed evidence of past reimplantation of one of the right ureters. Using a flexible ureteroscope, retrograde ureteroscopy was performed. Two tumors were found in the right upper ureter, one at the ureteropelvic junction and one below. Each was less than .5 cm in size. Using the rigid ureteroscope, the tumors were reached and, using a Bugbee electrode, fulguration of the tumors was carried out. Tissue that remained on the Bugbee electrode was retained and sent to pathology for microscopic study. All of the instruments were removed, and the patient was moved to recovery in good condition. She will receive Bactrim 1 b.i.d. for 10 days.

Case Explanation: The fulguration of the ureter would code to the root operation Destruction (0T568ZZ) in ICD-10-PCS. The approach would be via natural or artificial opening endoscopic because it was performed via an ureteroscopy. The procedure code would be repeated, because two tumors were fulgurated. See Coding Guideline B3.2.b.

Case Example #19

The following case is for dental extraction, which is coded to 23.09 in ICD-9-CM. The code descriptor for 23.09 is Extraction of other tooth and is categorized under category 23.0, Forceps extraction of tooth.

Case Description: The patient is a 25-year-old woman with moderate mental retardation who needs dental extractions for dental caries in the pulp and chronic apical periodontitis. She will have four upper and five lower teeth removed. She is being put under anesthesia because of her mental retardation. Prior to surgery the patient was instructed to stop the anticoagulant drug, Coumadin, she is taking and begin taking Lovenox instead. The patient has a history of mitral valve and aortic valve replacements and needs subacute bacterial endocarditis prophylaxis before the surgery. She is taking the anticoagulation therapy because of her past heart surgery. She also needed to be monitored for therapeutic anticoagulant drug levels prior to surgery. Management of the anticoagulation was completed in 2 days, and the patient had the simple dental extractions with forceps on day 3. The patient was allowed to return home on day 5 after the Coumadin was restarted on day 4 with no ill effects. The patient has follow-up appointments with the oral surgeon and the family physician in the next week.

Case Explanation: The forceps removal of the teeth would code to the root operation Extraction (0CDXXZ1, 0CDWXZ1) in ICD-10-PCS. There is documentation that multiple upper (four) and lower (five) teeth were removed. The seventh character (qualifier) identifies single (0), multiple (1) or all (2). In this case the removal was done with forceps. The patient's teeth could be seen in the mouth and the procedure was done with a forceps. This would meet the definition of Extraction. The patient was taken to surgery and given anesthesia because of her mental retardation. When teeth cannot be seen easily because they have broken off at the gum line or not come in yet, a surgical extraction may be required. In these cases the oral surgeon cuts and pulls back the gums. Pulling back the gum flap provides access to remove bone and/or a piece of the tooth. These surgical extractions would be coded to 23.19 in ICD-9-CM and may be coded to resection in ICD-10-PCS, depending on the intent of the procedure.

Case Example #20

The following case is for a suction dilation & curettage, which is coded to 69.09 in ICD-9-CM. The code descriptor for 69.09 is Other dilation and curettage and is categorized under category 69.0, Dilation and curettage of uterus.

Case Description: This 35-year-old female patient was scheduled for diagnostic dilation & curettage. After induction of general anesthesia, the patient was placed in the dorsal lithotomy position and appropriately prepped and draped. Successive dilators were placed until the cervix was adequate for insertion of the suction cannula. Suction cannula was placed and suction curettage performed with no residual endometrial lining. The tissue was sent to pathology to rule out endometrial cancer.

Case Explanation: The suction dilation & curettage (D&C) would code to the root operation Extraction (0U**D**B7ZX) in ICD-10-PCS. During the curettage (which means scraping) a uterine curette is inserted and the uterine wall scraped. Suction is often performed first so that the material can be sent for pathological examination. The dilation is inherent in the procedure and would not be separately coded. In order to do the curettage, the dilation is necessary to reach the procedure site. There was no documentation that an endoscope was used, so the approach would be via natural or artificial opening (7) and the qualifier is X for diagnostic.

Chapter 5

Medical and Surgical Section: Root Operations That Take Out Solids/ Fluids/Gases from a Body Part and Root Operations Involving Cutting or Separation Only

Root Operations That Take Out Solids/ Fluids/Gases from a Body Part

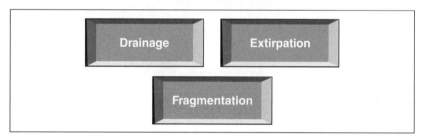

Drainage: 9

Definition	Taking or letting out fluids and/or gases from a body part
Explanation	The qualifier Diagnostic is used to identify drainage procedures that are biopsies
Examples	Thoracentesis, incision and drainage

The root operation Drainage is coded for both diagnostic and therapeutic drainage procedures. When drainage is accomplished by putting in a catheter, the device value Drainage Device is coded in the sixth character.

Additional Examples of Drainage Procedures

- Right hip arthrotomy with drain placement
- Diagnostic percutaneous paracentesis for ascites
- Incision and drainage of external perianal abscess

- Routine Foley catheter placement
- Laparoscopy with right ovarian cystotomy and drainage
- Laparotomy with hepatotomy and drain placement for liver abscess, left lobe
- Thoracentesis of left pleural effusion
- Percutaneous chest tube placement for right pneumothorax
- Urinary nephrostomy catheter placement
- Endoscopic drainage of right ethmoid sinus

Extirpation: C

Definition   Taking or cutting out solid matter from a body part

Explanation   The solid matter may be an abnormal byproduct of a biological function or a foreign body, or it may be imbedded in a body part or in the lumen of a tubular body part. The solid matter may or may not have been previously broken into pieces.

Examples   Thrombectomy, choledocholithotomy

Extirpation represents a range of procedures where the body part itself is not the focus of the procedure. Instead, the objective is to remove solid material such as a foreign body, thrombus, or calculus from the body part.

Additional Examples of Extirpation Procedures

- Percutaneous mechanical thrombectomy, right common interosseous artery
- Forceps removal of foreign body in the left nostril
- Foreign body removal, skin of right index finger
- De-clotting of arteriovenous dialysis graft
- Removal of foreign body, left cornea
- Esophagogastroscopy with removal of bezoar from stomach
- Transurethral cystoscopy with removal of bladder calculus
- Laparoscopy with excision of old suture from mesentery
- Incision and removal of right lacrimal duct calculus
- Non-incisional removal of intraluminal foreign body from vagina
- Open excision of retained foreign body, subcutaneous tissue of left foot

Fragmentation: F

Definition   Breaking solid matter in a body part into pieces

Explanation   The physical force (for example, manual, ultra-sonic) applied directly or indirectly is used to break the solid matter into pieces. The solid matter may be an abnormal byproduct of a biological function or a foreign body. The pieces of solid matter are not taken out.

Examples   Extracorporeal shockwave lithotripsy, transurethral lithotripsy

Fragmentation is coded for procedures to break up, but not remove, solid material such as a calculus or foreign body. This root operation includes both direct and extracorporeal Fragmentation procedures.

Additional Examples of Fragmentation Procedures

- Extracorporeal shockwave lithotripsy (ESWL), bilateral ureters
- Transurethral cystoscopy with fragmentation of bladder neck calculus
- Endoscopic retrograde cholangiopancreatography (ERCP) with lithotripsy of common bile duct stone
- Hysteroscopy with intraluminal lithotripsy of left fallopian tube calcification
- Thoracotomy with crushing of pericardial calcifications
- Extracorporeal shockwave lithotripsy (ESWL) of left kidney

Apply Knowledge to Transition from Coding in ICD-9-CM to ICD-10-PCS

Case Example #1

The following case is for an incision and drainage of a pilonidal cyst, which is coded to 86.03 in ICD-9-CM. The code descriptor for 86.03 is Incision of pilonidal sinus or cyst and is categorized under category 86.0, Incision of skin and subcutaneous tissue.

Case Description: A 20-year-old woman was scheduled for an outpatient procedure to treat a pilonidal cyst that had become abscessed. The procedure performed was an incision and drainage of the pilonidal sinus. The patient will continue to take oral antibiotics to resolve the infection. The patient was discharged home with a follow-up appointment in 7 days with the surgeon who performed the procedure.

Case Explanation: An incision and drainage procedure would code to the root operation Drainage (0H98XZZ) in ICD-10-PCS. A pilonidal cyst is a cyst that develops along the tailbone (coccyx) near the cleft of the buttocks. During this procedure the area is numbed with a local anesthetic and an incision is made over the infected area. Once the incision is made the pus is then drained. In this case a drainage device was not left at the operative site but if one was left the code is 0H98X0Z.

Case Example #2

The following case is for an insertion of a chest tube to drain fluid from the left pleural cavity. In ICD-9-CM this procedure would be coded to 34.04, Insertion of intercostal catheter for drainage and is categorized under category 34.0, Incision of chest wall and pleura. The code 34.04 would be coded for insertion of chest tube in either the right or left pleural cavity.

Case Description:

History: The patient is a 65-year-old man with stage 4 gastroesophageal junction carcinoma. He developed severe respiratory distress and was brought to the hospital emergency department and admitted. A large left pleural effusion was noted on CT scan and chest x-ray. A chest tube insertion was recommended to relieve the patient's respiratory failure caused by the pleural effusion, and the patient consented to the procedure.

Description of Procedure: The patient was in the supine position in the medical intensive care unit on propofol drip. His left anterior chest was prepped and draped. One percent Xylocaine was given, and a small incision was made. Using the hemostat, the chest cavity was entered and fluid was returned. Then using the trocar, the chest tube was placed in the superior portion of the left upper lobe. There was approximately 1000 ml of fluid returned. The patient tolerated the procedure well, and the chest tube was sewn in place. A follow-up chest x-ray confirmed good positioning of the tube, and a decrease in the amount of pleural effusion was noted.

Case Explanation: The correct root operation for this procedure is Drainage (0W9B30Z) as the objective of this procedure is to take out or drain the excess fluid from the left pleural cavity. During this procedure a chest tube was percutaneously inserted into the left pleural cavity and fluid was drained. 0W9930Z would be the correct ICD-10-PCS code if fluid was drained from the right pleural cavity.

Case Example #3

The following case is a lumbar puncture or spinal tap. In this instance, the spinal tap is diagnostic and codes to 03.31 in ICD-9-CM and is categorized under category 03.3, Diagnostic procedures on spinal cord and spinal canal structures. If a therapeutic spinal tap was performed the correct ICD-9-CM code is 03.09.

Case Description: A 20-year-old college student was brought to the emergency department complaining of a sudden onset of headache, fever, and stiffness with pain in the neck. He had been treated in the college health service center for an ear infection in the past week. After admission, the patient also complained of chest pain, fatigue, cough, and nausea. A lumbar puncture was performed and the findings were positive for meningitis. A chest x-ray revealed pneumonia. Sputum and spinal fluid cultures grew the pneumococcus organism (*Streptococcus pneumoniae.*) The physical examination also confirmed the presence of acute otitis media. The patient was treated with intravenous antibiotics for the infections. The discharge diagnoses written by the physician were pneumococcal meningitis with pneumococcal pneumonia and acute suppurative otitis media.

Case Explanation: A diagnostic lumbar puncture would code to the root operation Drainage (009Y3ZX) in ICD-10-PCS. During this procedure a needle is inserted into the lumbar subarachnoid space to withdraw cerebrospinal fluid. The seventh character of "X" indicates that this is a diagnostic procedure.

Case Example #4

The following case is for a percutaneous nephrostomy, which is coded to 55.03 in ICD-9-CM. The code descriptor for 55.03 is Percutaneous nephrostomy without fragmentation and is categorized under category 55.0, Nephrotomy and nephrostomy. ICD-9-CM does not differentiate whether the procedure is performed on the right or left kidney. If fragmentation had also been performed the correct code would be 55.04, Percutaneous nephrostomy with fragmentation.

Case Description: A 70-year-old male patient was admitted to the hospital with the diagnosis of left ureteral obstruction. Known to have a primary malignancy of the stomach that was surgically resected 6 months earlier, the patient was still receiving chemotherapy for the gastric malignancy. Outpatient testing showed evidence of ureteral obstruction, and the patient was admitted for evaluation and possible surgical treatment to relieve the obstruction and abate the symptoms it produced. A surgical consultation was obtained from a urologist and the patient consented to surgery. The urologist performed a percutaneous nephrostomy to relieve the obstruction that was caused by ureteral metastatic disease. Evidence of intra-abdominal metastasis was also found. The patient did not want further aggressive therapy and was discharged home to consider using hospice services.

Case Explanation: A percutaneous nephrostomy procedure would code to the root operation Drainage (0T**9**130Z) in ICD-10-PCS. During this procedure, the physician usually uses x-ray and/or ultrasound to locate the kidney and a needle is inserted through the skin and into the kidney. The nephrostomy catheter will then be inserted into the kidney. The nephrostomy catheter is placed to allow drainage. In this case the percutaneous nephrostomy was performed on the left kidney, if performed on the right kidney the ICD-10-PCS code would be 0T**9**030Z.

Case Example #5

The following case is for a thrombectomy of arteriovenous graft, which is coded to 39.49 in ICD-9-CM. The code descriptor for 39.49 is Other revision of vascular procedure and is categorized under category 39.4, Revision of vascular procedure. Code 39.49 is an "other specified" code in ICD-9-CM with multiple different vascular procedures being classified to this code.

Case Description: This 73-year-old woman was admitted to the hospital for pneumonia and on the third day of her hospitalization she was also found to have an occlusion of her left forearm arteriovenous graft.

A thrombectomy was recommended and the patient consented to the procedure. The patient was taken to the operating room and placed in the supine position. Her left arm was prepared and draped in the normal fashion. A transverse incision was made at the outflow tract of the basilic vein and the Gore-Tex graft anastomosis. A complete thrombectomy was performed. The area was fully irrigated with saline and heparin lock. There was satisfactory pulse through the graft and the incisions were closed with 3-0 Dexon and running 4-0 Prolene.

Case Explanation: The correct root operation for the thrombectomy is Extirpation (05**C**C0ZZ) as the objective of this procedure is to remove the thrombus in the left basilic vein. The fourth character of this code captures that the thrombus was removed or extirpated from the left basilic vein.

Case Example #6

The following case is for a removal of a foreign body lodged in the trachea, which is coded to 98.15. The code descriptor for 98.15 is Removal of intraluminal foreign body from trachea and bronchus without incision and is categorized under category 98.1, Removal of intraluminal foreign body from other sites without incision. This code is used for removal of a foreign body from both the trachea and the bronchus. A second procedure code of 31.42 is needed for the laryngoscope. If an incision was made in order to remove the foreign body from the trachea, the correct ICD-9-CM code is 31.3, Other incision of larynx or trachea.

Case Description: A 10-year-old choking on a small latex balloon is rushed from the amusement park to the emergency department. The balloon is lodged in the trachea just past the larynx and threatening to obstruct her breathing. The piece of latex balloon is carefully removed from the trachea by use of biopsy forceps through flexible fiberoptic laryngoscope following administration of topical anesthesia.

Case Explanation: The removal of a foreign body from the trachea would code to the root operation Extirpation (0B**C**18ZZ) in ICD-10-PCS. Unlike the ICD-9-CM code 98.15, code 0B**C**18ZZ is for removal of a foreign body from the trachea only. If a foreign body was removed from the bronchus then the fourth character of the code would have a different value. A secondary code for the laryngoscope is not necessary in ICD-10-PCS since the fifth character of the code captures that the procedure was performed "via natural or artificial opening endoscopic". If an incision was made in order to remove the foreign body from the trachea, the ICD-10-PCS code would be 0B**C**10ZZ.

Case #7

The following case is for a removal of bladder calculus via cystoscope, which is coded to 57.0 in ICD-9-CM. The code descriptor for 57.0 is Transurethral clearance of bladder and includes both drainage of the bladder without incision and removal of blood clot, calculus or foreign body without incision. This is categorized under category 57, Operations on urinary bladder. This code would be used to code both an extirpation and drainage of a calculus from the bladder or bladder neck.

Case Description: The patient was taken to the operating suite and placed in the dorsal lithotomy position, and then sterilely prepared and draped in the usual fashion. Cystoscope was inserted into the urethra; it was normal. The scope was then advanced into the bladder where a calculus was noted. The calculus was removed and the scope was then withdrawn. The patient was transferred to the recovery room in satisfactory condition.

Case Explanation: The removal of a calculus is coded to the root operation Extirpation (0T**C**B8ZZ) in ICD-10-PCS. Unlike the ICD-9-CM code 57.0, code 0T**C**B8ZZ is only for removal of a blood clot, calculus or foreign body from the bladder. If fluids had been drained from the bladder, Drainage, not Extirpation, would be the correct root operation.

Case Example #8

The following case is for an extracorporeal shockwave lithotripsy procedure. In ICD-9-CM this procedure would be coded to 98.51, Extracorporeal shockwave lithotripsy [ESWL] of the kidney, ureter and/or bladder and is categorized under category 98.5, Extracorporeal shockwave lithotripsy [ESWL].

Case Description: Under IV sedation, the patient was placed in the supine position. The stone in the upper right kidney was positioned at F2. The extracorporeal lithotripsy was started at 19 KV, which subsequently was increased to a maximum of 26 KV at 1,600 shocks. The stone was revisualized, and repositioning was done considering the transverse colon passing right anterior to the stone. Because the stone appeared to be in the same place after the repositioning, shocks were delivered. Apparent adequate fragmentation was obtained after a total of 2,400 shocks had been administered. The patient tolerated the procedure quite well.

Case Explanation: The root operation for this procedure is Fragmentation (0TF3XZZ) as the objective of this procedure is to break up, but not remove, the calculus located in the right kidney. During this procedure the patient reclines on a machine bed, which has a water-filled back support positioned behind the kidneys. Using x-ray or ultrasound imaging the stone(s) are located. High-energy sound waves pass through the patient's body and break the stone(s) into small pieces. These small pieces move through the urinary tract and out of the body. Unlike the ICD-9-CM code 98.51, code 0TF3XZZ is for fragmentation of stones in the right kidney only. If the stone was located either in the left kidney, bladder or ureter then the fourth character of the code would have a different value.

Root Operations Involving Cutting or Separation Only

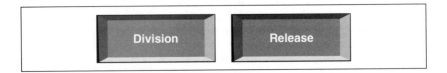

Division: 8

Definition   Cutting into a body part without draining fluids and/or gases from the body part in order to separate or transect a body part

Explanation   All or a portion of the body part is separated into two or more portions

Examples   Spinal cordotomy, osteotomy

The root operation Division is coded when the objective of the procedure is to cut into, transect, or otherwise separate all or a portion of a body part. When the objective is to cut or separate the area around a body part, the attachments to a body part, or between subdivisions of a body part that are causing abnormal constraint, then the root operation Release is coded instead.

Coding Guideline: B3.14 Release vs. Division

If the sole objective of the procedure is freeing a body part without cutting the body part, the root operation is Release. If the sole objective of the procedure is separating or transecting a body part, the root operation is Division.

> **Examples:**   Freeing a nerve root from surrounding scar tissue to relieve pain is coded to the root operation Release.
>
> Severing a nerve root to relieve pain is coded to the root operation Division.

Additional Examples of Division Procedures

- Open osteotomy of capitate, right hand
- Division of left Achilles tendon, percutaneous
- Left heart catheterization with division of bundle of His
- Sacral rhizotomy for pain control, percutaneous
- Anal sphincterotomy
- EGD with esophagotomy of esophagogastric junction

Release: N

Definition	Freeing a body part from an abnormal physical constraint by cutting or by use of force
Explanation	Some of the restraining tissue may be taken out but none of the body part is taken out
Examples	Adhesiolysis, carpal tunnel release

The objective of procedures represented in the root operation Release is to free a body part from abnormal constraint. Release procedures are coded to the body part being freed. The procedure can be performed on the area around a body part, on the attachments to a body part, or between subdivisions of a body part that are causing the abnormal constraint.

Coding Guideline: B3.13 Release Procedures

In the root operation Release, the body part value coded is the body part being freed and not the tissue being manipulated or cut to free the body part.

Example: Lysis of intestinal adhesions is coded to the specific intestine body part value.

Additional Examples of Release Procedures

- Left shoulder arthroscopy with coracoacromial ligament release
- Laparoscopy with freeing of bilateral ovaries and fallopian tubes
- Left open carpal tunnel release

- Incision of scar contracture, left elbow
- Open posterior tarsal tunnel release
- Manual rupture of left shoulder joint adhesions under general anesthesia
- Laparoscopy with lysis of peritoneal adhesions
- Mitral valvulotomy for release of fused leaflets, open
- Frenulotomy for treatment of tongue-tie syndrome

Apply Knowledge to Transition from Coding in ICD-9-CM to ICD-10-PCS

Case Example #1

The following case is for a left lateral sphincterotomy, which is coded to 49.51 in ICD-9-CM. The code descriptor for 49.51 is Left lateral anal sphincterotomy, and is categorized under category 49.5, Division of anal sphincter. ICD-9-CM does not differentiate the approach to performing the sphincterotomy with all approaches coding to 49.51. If a posterior anal sphincterotomy had been performed, the correct ICD-9-CM procedure code would be 49.52 instead of 49.51.

Case Description: A 35-year-old male was scheduled to have a left lateral sphincterotomy for treatment of a chronic anal fissure. The patient was taken to the operating room where a left lateral sphincterotomy was done at the 4 o'clock position using a percutaneous approach, dividing only the left internal sphincter using the #11 blade.

Case Explanation: A left lateral sphincterotomy would code to the root operation Division (0D8R3ZZ) in ICD-10-PCS. Sphincterotomy surgery is performed to allow the anal fissure or fistula to heal. During the procedure a small part of the anal sphincter muscle is cut to open the anal canal. This relieves the pressure and allows the fistula to heal. ICD-10-PCS, unlike ICD-9-CM, differentiates the approach to performing this procedure, such as open or percutaneous. The fifth character value will be different depending on the surgical approach.

Case Example #2

The following case is for a percutaneous cervical cordotomy, which is coded to 03.21 in ICD-9-CM. The code descriptor for 03.21 is Percutaneous chordotomy and is categorized under category 03.2, Chordotomy. ICD-9-CM does not differentiate between the different levels of the spine (that is, cervical, lumbar, thoracic) for cordotomies. Therefore all percutaneous cordotomies of any level of the spine are coded to 03.21. If a cordotomy is performed by a different type of approach such as open the correct code is 03.29, Other chordotomy.

Case Description: A 59-year-old patient was admitted to the hospital due to extremely severe pain as a result of adenocarcinoma of the prostate which has metastasized to the bone. The patient has been experiencing pain in the cervical area for the past 3–4 weeks with no relief from the usual treatments. A percutaneous cervical cordotomy was recommended and performed to provide the patient relief from the pain.

Case Explanation: The correct root operation for this procedure is Division (00**8**W3ZZ) as the objective of this procedure is to transect a body part by cutting into the body part without draining fluids and/or gases. Spinal cordotomies are surgical procedures that are used to alleviate recurring pain and sometimes are performed on patients experiencing severe pain due to cancer. During this procedure the spinal nerve roots within the spinal canal are surgically severed to relieve the pain. The fourth character of a spinal cordotomy procedure in ICD-10-PCS captures the level of the spine the procedure is being performed on (cervical, lumbar or thoracic).

Case Example #3

The following case is for a percutaneous lengthening tenotomy of the Achilles tendon, which is coded to 83.11 in ICD-9-CM. The code descriptor for 83.11 is Achillotenotomy, and this code is used for both percutaneous and open approaches to perform this procedure. Code 83.11 is categorized under category 83.1, Division of muscle, tendon, and fascia.

Case Description: The patient underwent a percutaneous tenotomy of his left Achilles tendon for correction of contracture of the Achilles tendon. During the procedure a thin blade was inserted through the skin to partially severe or cut the Achilles tendon.

Case Explanation: A percutaneous tenotomy of the Achilles tendon would code to the root operation Division (0L**8**P3ZZ) in ICD-10-PCS.

During this procedure, the tendon is severed in order to lengthen the tendon, allowing a muscle to return to its normal length and allowing the joint to straighten. Unlike the ICD-9-CM code 83.11, ICD-10-PCS differentiates the various approaches used to perform the procedure at the fifth character position.

Case Example #4

The following case is for lysis of adhesions of the small bowel, which is coded to 54.59 in ICD-9-CM. The code descriptor for 54.59 is Lysis of peritoneal adhesions and this code is used for freeing of adhesions of the following body parts or areas: biliary tract, intestines, liver, pelvic peritoneum, peritoneum, spleen and uterus. This is categorized under category 54.5, Lysis of peritoneal adhesions. If the lysis of peritoneal adhesions had been performed laparoscopically rather than open, 54.51 would be the correct ICD-9-CM code. An additional code of 99.77 would also be coded for the application of adhesion barrier substance.

Case Description:

History: The patient is an 85-year-old woman who lives independently with her husband in her own home and has been treated for hypothyroidism, hypertension, and dyslipidemia in the past. Medications for these conditions were continued during her hospital stay. Early this morning she awoke with acute onset of right flank pain. Her husband called 911 and she was brought to the emergency department of this hospital. On examination she was found in be in acute pain with a palpable mass in her abdominal area. Radiologic examination found dilated loops of small bowel trapped between the abdominal wall and the ascending colon and cecum. She was taken emergently to the operating room for a suspected small bowel obstruction.

Operative Findings: The procedure performed was an exploratory laparotomy and release of acute closed loop small-bowel obstruction due to adhesions by lysis of adhesions. Fortunately the bowel was viable and did not have to be resected.

Description of Procedure: After routine preparation, the patient was taken to the operating room. A midline incision was made through the scar of previous surgery, which was a hysterectomy. Supraumbilical extension of the scar was performed. Once the adhesions were taken down, the abdominal cavity was entered. One loop of small bowel was going through the defect created between the omentum and ascending colon and was trapped in that space. The adhesions were transected and the small bowel obstruction was released. The entire small bowel was mobilized and explored from the ligament of Treitz all the way to the ileocecal valve. The wound was irrigated. Hemostasis was obtained after lysis of adhesions that released the acute small bowel obstruction. Lap count and instrument count were correct. Seprafilm adhesion barrier substance was placed in the peritoneal cavity prior to closure. The fascia was closed with PDS loop. The skin was closed with skin stapler. A dressing was applied. The patient tolerated the procedure well under general anesthesia and was taken to the post-anesthesia recovery area in good condition.

Case Explanation: Lysis of small intestine adhesions would code to the root operation Release (0DN80ZZ) in ICD-10-PCS. Release is the correct root operation as the objective of a lysis procedure is to free or release a body part, in this case the small intestine, from abnormal constraint. Release procedures are coded to the body part being freed so in this case the correct body part is the small intestines. Unlike the ICD-9-CM code 54.59, ICD-10-PCS allows you to code the specific body part being released at the fourth character position. Similar to ICD-9-CM, an additional code is assigned for the application of adhesion barrier substance, 3E0M05Z.

Case Example #5

The following case is for a carpal tunnel release, which is coded to 04.43 in ICD-9-CM. The code descriptor for 04.43 is Release of carpal tunnel and is categorized under 04.4, Lysis of adhesions and decompression of cranial and peripheral nerves. ICD-9-CM does not differentiate the approach for performing the procedure. Therefore both open and arthroscopic carpal tunnel release procedures code to 04.43.

Case Description:

Preoperative Diagnosis: Carpal tunnel compression, left, severe

Postoperative Diagnosis: Carpal tunnel compression, left, severe

Operation: Left carpal tunnel release

Procedure: After successful axillary block was placed, the patient's left arm was prepared and draped in the usual sterile manner. Tourniquet was inflated. A curvilinear hypothenar incision was made and the palmaris retracted radially. The carpal tunnel and the transverse carpal ligament were then opened and completely freed in the proximal directions. It was noted to be severely tight in the palm with flattening and swelling of the median nerve. The carpal tunnel was opened distally in the hand and noted to be clear. The wound was then closed with 4-0 Dexon in subcuticular tissues. Sterile bulky dressing was applied and the patient was taken to the recovery room in satisfactory condition.

Case Explanation: A carpal tunnel release procedure would code to the root operation Release (01N50ZZ) in ICD-10-PCS. During a carpal tunnel release procedure, the transverse carpal ligament is cut, which releases the pressure on the median nerve and relieves the symptoms of the carpal tunnel syndrome. Since Release procedures are coded to the body part being freed, the body part value for this procedure would be the median nerve. Unlike the ICD-9-CM code 04.43, ICD-10-PCS provides specific codes for open versus percutaneous carpal tunnel release procedures.

Case Example #6

The following procedure is for a manual rupture of adhesive capsulitis (adhesions) of the left shoulder under general anesthesia, which is coded to 93.26 in ICD-9-CM. The code descriptor for 93.26 is Manual rupture of joint adhesions and is categorized under category 93.2, Other physical therapy musculoskeletal manipulation. ICD-9-CM does not provide separate codes to differentiate the specific joint being released from the adhesions. Therefore all manual rupture of joint adhesions are coded with 93.26.

Case Description:

History: The patient is a 56-year-old male who has been scheduled to undergo a manual rupture of the left shoulder under general anesthesia. The patient has extensive adhesive capsulitis of the left shoulder which has not responded to other aggressive treatment. The patient has been aggressively treated with a combination of anti-inflammatory medications, cortisone injections, and physical therapy. Despite therapy, the patient continues to have a significant loss of range of motion of his left shoulder in all directions and has decided to have surgery for the capsulitis. The patient also is being treated for hypertensive heart disease and type 1 diabetes mellitus.

Description of Procedure: The patient was placed on the operating table and general anesthesia was administered. The left shoulder was then carefully maneuvered through a full range of motion multiple times to release the adhesions. The patient was then extubated and taken to the recovery room in satisfactory condition.

Case Explanation: The correct root operation for this procedure is Release (0RNKXZZ) as the objective of this procedure is to release the left shoulder joint from abnormal constraint. In contrast to the ICD-9-CM code 93.26, ICD-10-PCS provides a separate and distinct code for each different joint. Examples of these distinct ICD-10-PCS codes are:

- Release right shoulder joint—0RNJXZZ
- Release left wrist joint—0RNPXZZ
- Release right metacarpocarpal joint—0RNSXZZ
- Release cervical vertebral joint—0RN1XZZ
- Release left elbow joint—0RNMXZZ

Chapter 6

Medical and Surgical Section: Root Operations That Put In/Put Back or Move Some/All of a Body Part

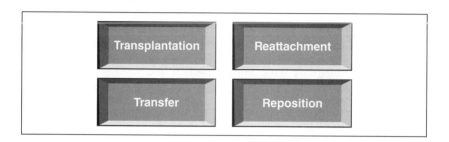

Transplantation: Y

Definition   Putting in or on all or a portion of a living body part taken from another individual or animal to physically take the place and/or function of all or a portion of a similar body part

Explanation   The native body part may or may not be taken out, and the transplanted body part may take over all or a portion of its function.

Examples   Kidney transplant, heart transplant

A small number of procedures is represented in the root operation Transplantation and includes only the body parts currently being transplanted. Qualifier values specify the genetic compatibility of the body part transplanted.

Coding Guideline: B3.16 Transplantation vs. Administration

Putting in a mature and functioning living body part taken from another individual or animal is coded to the root operation Transplantation.

Putting in autologous or nonautologous cells is coded to the Administration section.

> **Example:** Putting in autologous or nonautologous bone marrow, pancreatic islet cells, or stem cells is coded to the Administration section.

Coding Note: Bone marrow transplant procedures are coded in section 3 of ICD-10-PCS, Administration, to the Root Operation 2, Transfusion.

Additional Examples of Transplantation Procedures

- Liver transplant with donor matched liver
- Left lung transplant, open, using organ donor match
- Open transplant of large intestine, organ donor match
- Left kidney and pancreas transplant, open, organ bank transplant
- Orthotopic heart transplant using porcine heart, open

Reattachment: M

Definition   Putting back in or on all or a portion of a separated body part to its normal location or other suitable location

Explanation   Vascular circulation and nervous pathways may or may not be reestablished

Examples   Reattachment of hand, reattachment of avulsed kidney

Procedures coded to Reattachment include putting back a body part that has been cut off or avulsed. Nerves and blood vessels may or may not be reconnected in a Reattachment procedure.

Additional Examples of Reattachment Procedure

- Complex reattachment of left index finger
- Replantation of avulsed scalp

- Reattachment of severed left ear
- Reattachment of traumatic right gastrocnemius avulsion, open
- Reattachment of severed right hand
- Closed replantation of three avulsed teeth, upper jaw

Transfer: X

Definition	Moving, without taking out, all or a portion of a body part to another location to take over the function of all or a portion of a body part
Explanation	The body part transferred remains connected to its vascular and nervous supply
Examples	Tendon transfer, skin pedicle flap transfer

The root operation Transfer is used to represent procedures where a body part is moved to another location without disrupting its vascular and nervous supply. In the body systems that classify the subcutaneous tissue, fascia and muscle body parts, a qualifier is used to specify when more than one tissue layer was used in the transfer procedure, such as musculocutaneous flap transfer.

Body System Value

The body system value describes the deepest tissue layer in the flap. The qualifier can be used to describe the other tissue layers, if any, being transferred.

Additional Examples of Transfer Procedures

- Left foot open flexor digitorum brevis tendon transfer
- Endoscopic radial to median nerve transfer
- Skin transfer flap closure of complex open wound, right chest
- Right scalp advancement flap to right temple
- Transfer right index finger to right thumb position, open
- Fasciocutaneous flap closure of left upper arm, open
- Trigeminal to fascial nerve transfer, percutaneous endoscopic
- Left leg flexor digitorum longus tendon transfer, percutaneous endoscopic
- Right wrist palmaris longus tendon transfer, open

Reposition: S

Definition	Moving to its normal location or other suitable location all or a portion of a body part
Explanation	The body part is moved to a new location from an abnormal location, or from a normal location where it is not functioning correctly. The body part may or may not be cut out or off to be moved to the new location
Examples	Reposition of undescended testicle, fracture reduction

Reposition represents procedures for moving a body part to a new location. The range of Reposition procedures includes moving a body part to its normal location, or moving a body part to a new location to enhance its ability to function.

Coding Guideline: B3.15 Reposition for Fracture Treatment

Reduction of a displaced fracture is coded to the root operation Reposition and the application of a cast or splint in conjunction with the Reposition procedure is not coded separately. Treatment of a nondisplaced fracture is coded to the procedure performed.

> **Examples:** Putting a pin in a nondisplaced fracture is coded to the root operation Insertion. Casting of a nondisplaced fracture is coded to the root operation Immobilization in the Placement section.

Additional Examples of Reposition Procedures

- Open fracture reduction with internal fixation, left tibia and ulna
- Relocation of bilateral undescended testicle, percutaneous
- Open fracture reduction, displaced fracture of right distal humerus
- Closed reduction with percutaneous internal fixation of left femoral neck fracture
- Right knee arthroscopy with reposition of patellar ligament
- Open transposition of ulnar nerve
- Laparoscopy with gastropexy for malrotation

Apply Knowledge to Transition from Coding in ICD-9-CM to ICD-10-PCS

Case Example #1

The following case is for a right kidney transplantation, which is coded to 55.69 in ICD-9-CM. The code descriptor for 55.69 is Other kidney transplantation and both right and left kidney transplantations are classified to this code and is categorized under category 55.6, Transplant of kidney. An additional code is required in ICD-9-CM to identify the donor as follows: 00.93, transplant from cadaver; 00.92, transplant from live non-related donor; and 00.91, transplant from live related donor. If the documentation does not specify the relationship of the donor, then no additional code is used.

Case Description: The patient is a 46-year-old male with end stage renal disease and type 1 diabetes mellitus. The patient is being admitted for right kidney transplantation. The donated kidney is a donor match kidney from a non-related individual. The patient was taken to the OR and placed on the table in the supine position. The patient was given general anesthesia and the abdominal area was prepped and draped in the usual fashion. A catheter was then placed in the bladder. An incision was made in the flank of the patient's abdomen. The donor kidney was placed in the lower right side of the abdomen above the pelvic bone and below the existing, non-functioning right kidney. The kidney artery and vein of the donor kidney were then sutured to the patient's iliac artery and vein. Next the ureter of the donor kidney was connected to the patient's bladder. The patient's non-functioning right kidney was left in place. The patient tolerated the procedure and was sent to the recovery room in stable condition.

Case Explanation: A right kidney transplantation of a donor kidney from another individual would code to the root operation Transplantation (0TY00Z0) in ICD-10-PCS. If a left kidney transplantation was performed the code would be 0TY10Z0 instead of 0TY00Z0. The seventh character (qualifier) of the transplantation code captures information regarding the donor kidney, therefore an additional code is not required. The information captured by the seventh character is different from the information captured by the additional code in ICD-9-CM. The seventh character for this code captures if the donor kidney is allogenic,

syngeneic, or zooplastic. An allogenic donor organ is taken from different individuals of the same species. A syngeneic donor organ is taken
from an individual having identical genes, such as an identical twin.
A zooplastic donor organ is taken from an animal. Whether or not the
native kidney was or was not taken out does not affect the code selection
and you are not required to code an additional code for removal of the
patient's own kidney as required in ICD-9-CM.

Case Example #2

The following case is for an orthotropic heart transplant, which is coded
to 37.51 in ICD-9-CM. The code description for 37.51 is Heart transplantation and is categorized under category 37.5, Heart replacement
procedures. If the donor heart is from a cadaver then an additional code
of 00.93 is also required. Additionally, code 39.61 is coded because the
patient is placed on a heart-lung bypass machine during the procedure.
If a combined heart-lung transplantation was performed, code 33.6
would be used instead of 37.51.

Case Description: The patient is a 56-year-old male who is being
admitted for a heart transplantation. The donor heart is from an unre-
lated individual. The patient was taken to the OR and placed on the table
in the supine position. The patient was given general anesthesia and the
chest area was prepped and draped in the usual fashion. The patient was
placed on the heart-lung bypass machine. The chest cavity was then
opened. The patient's own diseased heart was removed except for the
back half of both upper chambers of the heart (atria). The donor heart
was then trimmed and sewn to fit the remaining parts of the patient's
old heart. The donor heart's left atrium was then sewn onto the recipi-
ent's left atrium. Next the donor heart's right atrium was sewn onto the
superior and inferior vena cava. The heart-lung bypass machine was
removed, the incision was closed and the patient was taken to the recovery room in satisfactory condition.

Case Explanation: The correct root operation for this procedure is
Transplantation (02YA0Z0) because the objective of this procedure is put
in a living body part taken from another individual to take the place of
the function of a similar body part. The seventh character (qualifier) of
the transplantation code captures information regarding the donor heart
therefore an additional code is not required. The information captured

by the seventh character is different from the information captured by the additional code in ICD-9-CM. The seventh character for this code captures if the donor heart is allogenic, syngeneic, or zooplastic. An allogenic donor organ is taken from different individuals of the same species. A syngeneic donor organ is taken from an individual having identical genes, such as an identical twin. A zooplastic donor organ is taken from an animal. The removal of the patient's diseased heart is included in the Transplantation code. Similar to ICD-9-CM, additional codes are required for the heart-lung bypass machine (5A**1**221Z, 5A**1**935Z). In code 5A1035Z, the presumption was made that this is less than 24 consecutive hours (fifth character 3). Other choices are: 24–96 consecutive hours, or greater than 96 consecutive hours.

Case Example #3

In the following case the patient has a reattachment of his right index finger, which is coded to 84.22 in ICD-9-CM. The code description for 84.22 is Finger reattachment and this code is used for reattachment of the right or left index, middle, ring or little finger. If the reattachment had been of the right or left thumb the code is 84.21 instead of 84.22. This is categorized under category 84.2, Reattachment of extremity.

Case Description:

History: A 25-year-old male was brought to the Emergency Room with a traumatic amputation of the right index finger. The patient was working on remodeling the family room of his home when he accidently severed the right index finger with a circular saw. His wife accompanied him and has the severed finger. The patient was taken directly to the OR for reattachment of the severed finger.

Description of Procedure: After administration of general anesthesia, the patient was prepped and draped in the normal fashion. There were circumferential lacerations about the finger, save for a cutaneous bridge and ulnar vascular pedicle present at the PIP level. Nonviable bony fragments were removed and then the distal portion of the PIP joint was reshaped with removal of cartilage using double-rongeurs. It was noted that the fractures through the proximal phalanx extended longitudinally. Stabilization was then carried out with 0.062 K-wire brought down through the distal finger, out through the fingertip, and then back into the proximal phalanx centrally.

The A2 pulley was restored, using figure of eight interrupted sutures of 4-0 Vicryl, reapproximating the flexor tendons. The extensor mechanisms and tendons were repaired using 4-0 Vicryl, and anchored to the periosteum on the middle phalanx. The skin was then trimmed and lacerations were closed with Prolene. The patient was then taken to the recovery room in satisfactory condition.

Case Explanation: The correct root operation for this procedure is Reattachment (0X**M**N0ZZ) as the objective of this procedure is to put back on the separated (right index finger) body part to its normal location. Unlike ICD-9-CM, ICD-10-PCS does provide specific codes depending on the finger being reattached. The fourth character of the code captures the specific finger: right index finger, left index finger, right middle finger, left middle finger, right ring finger, left ring finger, right little finger, or left little finger.

Case Example #4

The following case is for a rotational advancement flap skin graft of the right upper arm, which is coded to 86.74 in ICD-9-CM. The code descriptor for 86.74 is Attachment of pedicle or flap graft to other sites and is categorized under category 86.7, Pedicle grafts or flaps. ICD-9-CM does not differentiate the site of the graft; therefore, all pedicle or flap grafts are coded to 86.74 except for the hand, which is coded to 86.73. Additionally, the following types of grafts are categorized to this code: advanced flap, double pedicle flap, pedicle graft, rotating flap, sliding flap, and tube graft.

Case Description: The patient is scheduled for an advancement flap skin graft for a 10-square centimeter defect of the right upper arm. The patient was placed on the operating table in the prone position with the upper arm prepped and draped in sterile fashion. Utilizing 1 percent Xylocaine with epinephrine, a block of the site was performed. Undermining over the fascial level of the right upper arm was performed with rotation flaps, elevated into position and sutured deeply at the fascial level with #5-0 PDS interrupted, #6-0 PDS, superficial dermis, and #6-0 PDS running intracuticular on the skin. Total area of the graft was 10.0 square centimeters.

Case Explanation: An advancement flap skin graft of the upper right arm would code to the root operation Transfer (0H**X**BXZZ) in ICD-

10-PCS. During an advancement flap skin graft the body part (skin) is moved to another location without disrupting its vascular and nervous supply. Unlike ICD-9-CM, ICD-10-PCS does provide different codes dependent upon the location and laterality of the advancement flap skin graft. The site of the procedure is captured with the fourth character (body part).

Case Example #5

Code only the Medical and Surgical Section procedure.

The following case is for a closed reduction with internal fixation of fractures of the radius and ulna, which is coded to 79.12 in ICD-9-CM. The code descriptor for code 79.12 is Closed reduction of radius and ulna fractures with internal fixation and is categorized under category 79, Reduction of fracture and dislocation. This code is used for closed reduction with internal fixation of both radius and ulna fractures.

Case Description:

History: The patient is an 11-year-old boy who was riding his bicycle yesterday in front of his home and fell. Because of severe wrist pain, he was seen in the emergency department. X-rays confirmed a displaced right distal radius and ulna fracture. The emergency department physician placed the patient in a splint, and he has returned this morning to be admitted for follow-up care and treatment. He denies any head or neck injury or loss of consciousness. His mother witnessed the fall and confirms he did not appear to hit his head or suffer any other injury except for the right wrist.

Description of Procedure: The patient was taken to the operating room and placed supine on the table with all of his extremities adequately padded. The patient was given laryngeal mask anesthesia. The splint was removed from the right upper extremity and a closed reduction was performed. The fractures were found to reduce. Fluoroscopy was used to view the fractures in multiplanar views. Given the nature of the fracture pattern, it was deemed appropriate to pin the radius and ulna to increase stability. Two K wires were then placed percutaneously under direct fluoroscopic guidance across each fracture site. The growth plate was avoided. The fractures and pins were then visualized in multiplanar fluoroscopy and the fractures and pins were noted to be in good position. The pins were bent and cut. Final films were obtained. Sterile dressings followed by a sugar tong-type of splint were then applied. The patient tolerated the procedure well, was awakened in the operating room, and was taken to recovery. There were no complications of this procedure.

Case Explanation: The correct root operation for this procedure is Reposition (0P**S**H34Z and 0P**S**K34Z) as the objective of this procedure is to move the radius and ulna back to their normal location. The radius and ulna each have their own distinct body part value in ICD-10-PCS; therefore two codes are required to code this procedure. The sixth character (device) captures the internal fixation device.

Case Example #6

Case Description: The following case is a left orchiopexy, which is coded to 62.5 in ICD-9-CM. The code descriptor for 62.5 is Orchiopexy and is categorized to category 62, Operations on testes. ICD-9-CM does not differentiate orchiopexy procedures by the operative approach. Therefore, open, percutaneous, and percutaneous endoscopic orchiopexy all code to 62.5. Additionally, ICD-9-CM does not differentiate whether the procedure is performed on the right or left testicle or both testes.

History: This 2-year-old male has been scheduled for left orchiopexy for an undescended testicle. The patient is otherwise in good health. Both parents consented to the surgery and the patient was taken to the operating room.

Description of Procedure: The patient was brought to the operating room and placed supine on the operating table. Following the adequate induction of general anesthesia, an incision was made in the inguinal region and dissection carried down to the pelvic cavity, where the left testis was located and mobilized. The spermatic cord was located and freed from surrounding tissue, and its length judged to be sufficient. A 1.5-cm incision was made in the scrotum and a pouch created in the usual fashion. The left testicle was mobilized down through the inguinal canal into the scrotum, and stitched into place. The incisions were closed in layers and the patient was taken to the recovery room in satisfactory condition.

Case Explanation: An orchiopexy is categorized to the root operation Reposition (0V**S**B0ZZ) in ICD-10-PCS. The fifth character of the code differentiates the approach to reach the operative site and the fourth character identifies whether the procedure was performed on the left or right testicle or both testicles (bilateral).

Case Example #7

In the following case the patient had a closed reduction of his dislocated right shoulder, which is coded to 79.71 in ICD-9-CM. The code descriptor for 79.71 is Closed reduction of dislocation of shoulder and is categorized under category 79, Reduction of fracture and dislocation. Code 79.71 would be used whether the surgical approach was percutaneous, percutaneous endoscopic, or external. If an open reduction has been performed, the code would be 79.81 instead of 79.71. ICD-9-CM does not differentiate laterality; therefore, 79.71 is coded for both right and left shoulder closed dislocation reduction.

Case Description: The patient is a 30-year-old man who comes to the emergency department complaining of joint pain in his right shoulder. The patient, who was a state champion wrestler during his college years, reports that his shoulder has dislocated on several occasions since college when he had several traumatic dislocations of the same shoulder. On this occasion, the patient was lifting a box overhead to place on a shelf in his garage. X-rays were taken to examine the shoulder. The ED physician is unable to reduce the dislocation on the initial attempt. With light intravenous sedation, the physician completes a closed reduction of shoulder dislocation. The physician wrote chronic recurrent dislocation of right shoulder and traumatic arthritis of the right shoulder as the final diagnosis on the ED record.

Case Explanation: The correct root operation for a closed reduction of a dislocated shoulder is Reduction (0R**S**JXZZ) as the objective of this procedure is to move the shoulder back to its normal position. ICD-10-PCS does provide distinct codes for the different surgical approaches; open, percutaneous, percutaneous endoscopic, and external. Additionally, ICD-10-PCS differentiates a shoulder reduction on the right (0RSJXZZ) versus the left (0RSKXZZ).

Case Example #8

The following case is for an open reduction with internal fixation (ORIF) of a humeral shaft fracture, which is coded to 79.31 in ICD-9-CM. The code descriptor for 79.31 is Open reduction of fracture of humerus with internal fixation which is categorized under category 79, Reduction of fracture and dislocation. ICD-9-CM does not differentiate laterality; therefore, ORIF of both the right and left humerus would code to this code. Additionally, the portion of the humerus that is fractured is not differentiated with this code and both ORIF of the head and the shaft of the humerus are coded with 79.31. Lastly, whether the physician used an internal fixation device versus an intramedullary fixation device is not differentiated in code 79.31.

Case Description:

History: The patient is a 50-year-old female who fell down the icy front steps of her house and sustained an injury to her left upper arm. X-ray of her left arm revealed a displaced fracture of the shaft of the humerus. She also hit her head on the concrete step and suffered a slight concussion but no loss of consciousness. The patient was admitted and taken to surgery for an open reduction with internal fixation of a displaced fracture of the shaft of the left humerus.

Description of Procedure: The patient was anesthetized and prepped with Betadine. Sterile drapes were applied, and the pneumatic tourniquet was inflated around the left arm. An incision was made in the area above the fracture, and this was carried through subcutaneous tissue, and the fracture site was easily exposed. Inspection revealed the fragment to be rotated in two planes about 90 degrees. It was possible to manually reduce this quite easily, and the judicious manipulation resulted in an almost anatomic reduction. This was fixed with two pins driven across the humerus. These pins were cut off below skin level. The wound was closed with some plain catgut suture subcutaneously and 5-0 nylon in the skin. Dressings were applied to the patient and tourniquet released. A long arm cast was applied.

Case Explanation: An open reduction with internal fixation for a displaced fracture of the shaft of the left humerus would code to the root operation Reposition (0PSG04Z) in ICD-10-PCS. Unlike ICD-9-CM, ICD-10-PCS differentiates both laterality (right versus left) and the portion of the humerus (head versus shaft) the procedure is performed on. Additionally, the sixth character of the code specifies whether the device was an internal fixation device or an intramedullary fixation device.

Chapter 7

Medical and Surgical Section: Root Operations That Alter the Diameter/Route of a Tubular Body Part

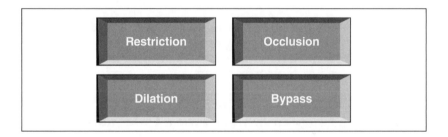

Restriction: V

Definition	Partially closing an orifice or the lumen of a tubular body part
Explanation	The orifice can be a natural orifice or an artificially created orifice
Examples	Esophagogastric fundoplication; cervical cerclage

The root operation Restriction is coded when the objective of the procedure is to narrow the diameter of a tubular body part or orifice. Restriction includes either intraluminal or extraluminal methods for narrowing the diameter.

When studying this root operation, it is helpful to review procedure methodology. Table 7.1 provides additional information on the two examples provided above.

Table 7.1. Procedure and technique

Procedure	Technique
Esophagogastric fundoplication	The gastric fundus of the stomach is wrapped (or plicated) around the lower end of the esophagus, thus reinforcing the esophageal sphincter closing function. The surgery actually strengthens the valve between the esophagus and the stomach and it is used to treat gastric reflux disease. In other words, the esophagogastric junction is restricted. A common technique used in fundoplication is the Nissen. Sometimes the procedure needs to be repeated due to symptoms. If Marlex mesh is used in the repeat procedure, then the root operation is not Restriction but rather Supplement.
Cervical cerclage	This procedure is done for an incompetent cervix. The cerclage is used to prevent early changes in a woman's cervix, thus preventing premature labor. During the procedure, a band of strong thread is stitched around the cervix.

Additional Examples of Restriction Procedures

- Thoracotomy with banding of left pulmonary artery with extraluminal device
- Restriction of thoracic duct with intraluminal stent
- Craniotomy with clipping of cerebral aneurysm
- Non-incisional, transnasal placement of restrictive stent in lacrimal duct

Because intraluminal or extraluminal clips are frequently used to accomplish the objectives of this procedure, careful review of the operative report is required. Research on the procedure technique may also be helpful. For example in a craniotomy with the clipping of the cerebral aneurysm, a clip is placed lengthwise on the outside wall of the widened portion of the vessel, so this would be considered an extraluminal device. In this procedure the neurosurgeon uses a microscope to isolate the blood vessel that feeds the aneurysm and places the small, metal, clothespin-like clip on the aneurysm's neck, thus halting the blood supply. This clip remains in the patient to prevent the risk of future bleeding.

Occlusion: L

Definition   Completely closing an orifice or the lumen of a
tubular body part

Explanation   The orifice can be a natural orifice or an
artificially created orifice

Examples   Fallopian tube ligation; ligation of inferior vena
cava

The root operation Occlusion is coded when the objective of the procedure is to close off a tubular body part or orifice. Occlusion includes
both intraluminal and extraluminal methods of closing off the body
part. Division of the tubular body part prior to closing it is an integral
part of the Occlusion procedure.

A fallopian tube ligation involves severing and sealing the tubes
to prevent pregnancy. There are several different ways to accomplish
this—such as with sutures, clips, or rings. If the procedure is performed
with electrocoagulation or cauterization, it is coded to Destruction, not
Occlusion.

The ligation of the inferior vena cava is performed to prevent recurrent pulmonary emboli due to venous thrombosis in the lower extremities or pelvis, or it may be done as a result of trauma.

Coding Guideline: B3.12 Occlusion vs. Restriction for Vessel Embolization Procedures

If the objective of an embolization procedure is to completely close
a vessel, the root operation Occlusion is coded. If the objective of an
embolization procedure is to narrow the lumen of a vessel, the root
operation Restriction is coded.

Examples: 1. Tumor embolization is coded to the root operation
Occlusion, because the objective of the procedure is to
cut off the blood supply to the vessel.

2. Embolization of a cerebral aneurysm is coded to the
root operation Restriction, because the objective of
the procedure is not to close off the vessel entirely,
but to narrow the lumen of the vessel at the site of the
aneurysm where it is abnormally wide.

Research on embolization may be required to gain additional information. The purpose of an embolization is to prevent blood flow to an area of the body. It is used during hemorrhage (for example, arteriovenous (AV) malformation, cerebral aneurysms, GI bleeding, epistaxis, postpartum hemorrhage). The procedure has other uses, such as in the treatment of tumors and disorders of the portal vein. An artificial embolus is introduced (coils, particles, foam, plugs) with some of the common agents used: sclerosing agents, ethanol, Gelfoam. In order to code occlusions and restrictions correctly, one must know if it is complete or partial, and physician documentation or additional physician query is essential.

Additional Examples of Occlusion Procedures

- Uterine artery embolization (completely closing the vessel)
- Ligation of esophageal vein
- Complete embolization of internal carotid-cavernous fistula
- Suture ligation of failed AV graft of brachial artery
- Complete embolization of vascular supply of intracranial meningioma

Dilation: 7

Definition	Expanding an orifice or the lumen of a tubular body part
Explanation	The orifice can be a natural orifice or an artificially created orifice. Accomplished by stretching a tubular body part using intraluminal pressure or by cutting part of the orifice or wall of the tubular body part
Examples	Percutaneous transluminal angioplasty (PTA), percutaneous transluminal coronary angioplasty (PTCA)

The root operation Dilation is coded when the objective of the procedure is to enlarge the diameter of a tubular body part or orifice. Dilation includes both intraluminal and extraluminal methods of enlarging the diameter. A device placed to maintain the new diameter is an integral part of the Dilation procedure, and is coded to a sixth-character device value in the Dilation procedure code.

During PTAs and PTCAs the narrowed or obstructed blood vessel is mechanically widened. Typically a collapsed balloon on a guide wire (balloon catheter) is passed into the narrowed locations and then inflated. The balloon crushes the fatty deposits, and then the balloon is collapsed and withdrawn. When a device is placed, it is coded to the sixth-character, and device values are:

- Drug-eluting intraluminal device
- Intraluminal device
- Radioactive intraluminal device

Coding Guideline: B4.4. Coronary Arteries

The coronary arteries are classified as a single body part that is further specified by number of sites treated and not by name or number of arteries. Separate body part values are used to specify the number of sites treated when the same procedure is performed on multiple sites in the coronary arteries.

Examples: Angioplasty of two distinct sites in the left anterior descending coronary artery with placement of two stents is coded as Dilation of Coronary Arteries, Two Sites, with Intraluminal Device.

Angioplasty of two distinct sites in the left anterior descending coronary artery, one with stent placed and one without, is coded separately as Dilation of Coronary Artery, One Site with Intraluminal Device, and Dilation of Coronary Artery, One Site with no device.

Additional Examples of Dilation Procedures

- ERCP with balloon dilation of common bile duct
- Cystoscopy with intraluminal dilation of bladder neck stricture
- Dilation of old anastomosis of femoral artery
- Dilation upper esophageal stricture using Bougie sound
- PTA brachial artery stenosis
- Transnasal dilation and stent placement lacrimal duct
- Hysteroscopy with balloon dilation of fallopian tubes
- Tracheoscopy with intraluminal dilation of tracheal stenosis
- Cystoscopy with dilation of ureteral stricture, with stent placement

Bypass: 1

Definition   Altering the route of passage of the contents of a
                   tubular body part

Explanation   Rerouting contents of a body part to a downstream
                   area of the normal route, to a similar route and
                   body part, or to an abnormal route and dissimilar
                   body part. Includes one or more anastomoses,
                   with or without the use of a device

Examples   Coronary artery bypass, colostomy formation

Bypass is coded when the objective of the procedure is to reroute
the contents of a tubular body part. The range of Bypass procedures
includes normal routes such as those made in coronary artery bypass
procedures, and abnormal routes such as those made in colostomy formation procedures.

Coding Guideline: B3.6a Bypass Procedures

Bypass procedures are coded by identifying the body part bypassed
"from" and the body part bypassed "to." The fourth character body part
specifies the body part bypassed from, and the qualifier specifies the
body part bypassed to.

> **Example:**   Bypass from stomach to jejunum, stomach is the body part
> and jejunum is the qualifier.

Coding Guideline: B3.6b

Coronary arteries are classified by number of distinct sites treated, rather
than number of coronary arteries or anatomic name of a coronary artery
(e.g., left anterior descending). Coronary artery bypass procedures are
coded differently than other bypass procedures as described in the previous guideline. Rather than identifying the body part bypassed from,
the body part identifies the number of coronary artery sites bypassed to,
and the qualifier specifies the vessel bypassed from.

> **Example:**   Aortocoronary artery bypass of one site on the left anterior
> descending coronary artery and one site on the obtuse mar-
> ginal coronary artery is classified in the body part axis of

classification as two coronary artery sites and the qualifier
specifies the aorta as the body part bypassed from.

Coding Guideline: B3.6c

If multiple coronary artery sites are bypassed, a separate procedure is
coded for each coronary artery site that uses a different device and/or
qualifier.

> **Example:** Aortocoronary artery bypass and internal mammary
> coronary artery bypass are coded separately.

Coding Guideline: B3.9. Excision for Graft

If an autograft is obtained from a different body part in order to complete the objective of the procedure, a separate procedure is coded.

> **Example:** Coronary bypass with excision of saphenous vein graft,
> excision of saphenous vein is coded separately.

Coding Note: An autograft is tissue or organ transferred into a
new position in the body of the same individual. Synonyms are:
autotransplant, autogeneic graft, autologous graft, autoplastic graft.
(Stedman's Electronic Medical Dictionary).

Additional Examples of Bypass Procedures

- Aorto-bifemoral bypass
- Gastric bypass with Roux-en-Y limb to jejunum
- Temporal artery to intracranial artery bypass using Gore-Tex
  graft
- Tracheostomy formation with tracheostomy tube placement
- Percutaneous in-situ coronary venous arterialization (PICVA)
  of single coronary artery
- Femoral-popliteal artery bypass
- Shunting of intrathecal cerebrospinal fluid to peritoneal cavity
  using synthetic shunt
- Urinary diversion, ureter, using ileal conduit to skin
- Pleuroperitoneal shunt, pleural cavity, using synthetic device

Apply Knowledge to Transition from Coding in ICD-9-CM to ICD-10-PCS

Case Example #1

The following case is for a laparoscopic gastric restrictive procedure, which is coded to 44.95 in ICD-9-CM. The code descriptor for 44.95 is Laparoscopic gastric restrictive procedure and is categorized under category 44.9, Other operations on stomach.

Case Description: The patient is a 27-year-old man who is admitted for laparoscopic bariatric surgery for morbid obesity. The patient currently weighs 200 lbs over his ideal body weight with a body mass index of 54. In the past 10 years he has lost and gained back more than 100 lbs, but now suffers from several major health conditions that require more aggressive management of his obesity. He has a strong family history of morbid obesity. It occurs in his parents, two sisters, and one brother. In the past 10 years, he has been treated for essential hypertension, dyslipidemia, obstructive sleep apnea, gallstone pancreatitis, type 2 diabetes, and osteoarthritis localized to his knees. He has had repeated failures of other therapeutic approaches to losing weight and has been cleared by a psychiatrist who could find no psychopathology that would make him ineligible for this procedure. His HMO has approved payment for the surgery. The patient underwent a laparoscopic gastric restrictive procedure with an adjustable gastric band and port insertion. The patient had an uneventful postoperative recovery in the hospital and was discharged for follow-up in the office. During this hospital stay, the conditions of hypertension, dyslipidemia, type 2 diabetes, and osteoarthritis localized to the knees were also treated.

Case Explanation: The restrictive procedure is coded to the root operation Restriction (0DV64CZ) in ICD-10-PCS. In this procedure, the gastric band device is placed around the upper part of the stomach, resulting in a pouch that reduces the capacity of the stomach. The band is adjustable, prolonging the efficacy of the procedure. The sixth character in the ICD-10-PCS code (C) identifies the extraluminal device.

Case Example #2

In the following case, only the tubal ligation will be discussed.

The following case is for a tubal ligation, which is coded to 66.31 in ICD-9-CM. The code descriptor for 66.31 is Other bilateral ligation and crushing of fallopian tubes, and is categorized under category 66.3, Other bilateral destruction or occlusion of fallopian tubes. In ICD-9-CM a distinction is made between endoscopic and other procedures, and between ligation and crushing and ligation and division of the fallopian tubes.

Case Description: The patient was admitted to the hospital from the obstetrician's office at 38 and $^3/_7$ weeks gestation. She came to the office today complaining of not feeling well and noticing a lack of fetal movement over the past day or two. She had been in the office 3 days ago and the baby was reactive. The biophysical profile in the office today was 6/8 with no breathing movement. The nonstress test was reactive. The patient also has severe iron deficiency anemia of pregnancy and hypertension complicating her pregnancy. She desires a tubal ligation during this delivery for her grand multiparity. She is 38 years old and gravida 6, para 3, AB 2 with an estimated date of delivery of June 30. She has had two previous cesarean deliveries, one in 1995 and one in 2005. Her oldest child was delivered vaginally in 1993. Because of the decreased fetal movement, a repeat low cesarean delivery was performed. A bilateral tubal ligation was also performed by ligation and crushing. Delivered at 4:55 p.m. was a 6 pound, 2 ounce live female infant with Apgar scores of 7 and 8. The patient had an uneventful recovery from the delivery, was continued on her medications for anemia and gestational hypertension, and asked to return to the office in 2 weeks. Mother and daughter were discharged home together on post-op day 3.

Case Explanation: A fallopian tube ligation would code to the root operation Occlusion (0UL70ZZ) in ICD-10-PCS. The approach selected would be Open because this procedure was done during a cesarean delivery. The usual manner for performing the procedure is laparoscopically. The crushing is part of the technique used to ligate the tube. There was no documentation that a clip or device was used.

Case Example #3

In the following case only the angioplasty will be discussed.

The following case is for a coronary angioplasty of the LAD with insertion of a non-drug-eluting stent, which is coded to 00.66 in ICD-9-CM. The code descriptor for 00.66 is Percutaneous transluminal coronary angioplasty [PTCA] or coronary artherectomy and is categorized under category 00.6, Procedures on blood vessels. The approach for this procedure is percutaneous according to the documentation. Further, in ICD-9-CM several other codes must be assigned in a code cluster to completely code this procedure. They are:

- 00.40, Procedure on single vessel
- 00.45, Insertion of one vascular stent
- 36.06, Insertion of non-drug-eluting coronary artery stent(s)

Any intracoronary artery thrombolytic infusion documented would also be coded.

Case Description: The patient is a 70-year-old man who was admitted by his cardiologist with the diagnosis of acute coronary syndrome. The patient had not had coronary angioplasty or coronary bypass surgery in the past. The patient consented to and underwent a diagnostic left heart cardiac catheterization and coronary arteriography by Judkins technique, which showed extensive arteriosclerotic coronary occlusion of the left anterior descending (LAD). Other vessels also had minor coronary artery disease. Prior to the procedure, the patient understood there was the possibility that he would require a coronary stent placement to which he also consented. Following completion of the diagnostic catheterization, the physician performed a coronary angioplasty of the LAD with the insertion of one non-drug-eluting coronary stent into the LAD. The physician's final diagnosis was "acute coronary syndrome due to arteriosclerotic coronary artery disease." The patient was discharged for follow-up evaluation and possible cardiac rehabilitation therapy.

Case Explanation: A PTCA of the coronary artery would code to the root operation Dilation (02703DZ) in ICD-10-PCS. Review of the guidelines related to coronary arteries is in order. Coronary arteries are classified as a single body part that is further specified by the number of sites treated and not by the name or number of arteries. In this case, only one site was treated. Further, only one stent (non-drug-eluting) was inserted, so only one code is assigned. The ICD-10-PCS code is the only one required for the PTCA since the number of arteries, the stent, and the type of stent can be identified in one code. No code cluster is needed in ICD-10-PCS. Percutaneous approach (3) is selected for this procedure.

Coronary angioplasty is done to open blocked or narrowed coronary arteries. Other names for this procedure are percutaneous transluminal coronary angioplasty (PTCA) or balloon angioplasty. During the procedure a balloon catheter is inserted into the coronary artery and positioned in the blockage. Then the balloon is expanded. This expansion pushes the plaque against the artery wall and relieves the blockage. If a stent is inserted, the stent is wrapped around the deflated balloon catheter before insertion, and then when inflated the stent expands and attaches to the artery wall. This provides support to the wall, and helps reduce the risk of the artery becoming narrowed subsequently (National Heart Lung and Blood Institute n.d.)

When coding this procedure, other procedures performed (diagnostic left heart cardiac catheterization and coronary arteriography) would also be coded.

Case Example #4

In the following case only the coronary artery bypass will be discussed.

The following case is for a triple coronary artery bypass graft, which is coded to 36.13 in ICD-9-CM. The code descriptor for 36.13 is Aortocoronary bypass of three coronary arteries and is categorized under category 36.1, Bypass anastomosis for heart revascularization. The vein graft harvesting is considered to be integral to the CABG in ICD-9-CM and is not coded separately.

Case Description: A 60-year-old male patient was admitted to the hospital with stable angina, which was continued under treatment. He underwent a combined right and left heart cardiac catheterization with coronary angiography, Judkins technique, and was determined to have significant atherosclerotic heart disease. Triple coronary artery bypass surgery was recommended for the 80% to 90% occlusion found in three native coronary vessels. The patient was also treated for type 2 diabetes that has been well controlled. With counseling and upon consent, the patient was scheduled for open heart surgery. An open triple coronary artery bypass graft, using greater saphenous veins from the leg (harvested laparoscopically), was performed on the left anterior descending, the circumflex, and the diagonal arteries. This was done using extracorporeal circulation.

Case Explanation: An aortocoronary bypass is coded to the root operation Bypass (02**1**209W) in ICD-10-PCS.

Coronary arteries are classified by number of distinct sites treated, rather than number of coronary arteries or anatomic name of a coronary artery. The fourth character for body part identifies the number of coronary artery sites bypassed to (2) and the seventh character for qualifier specifies the vessel bypassed from (W). The aorta is identified as the origin of the bypass. The sixth character of device is identified as autologous venous tissue (9) because this is tissue transferred into a new position in the body of the same individual. If multiple coronary artery sites are bypassed, a separate procedure is coded for each coronary artery site that uses a different device and/or qualifier. In this case, only one code is assigned because the device and qualifier do not change.

If as part of a procedure, an autograft is obtained from a different Body Part, a separate procedure is coded, so the saphenous vein graft would be coded to the root operation Excision (06BQ4ZZ).

When coding this case in ICD-10-PCS, other codes would also be assigned (combined right and left heart cardiac catheterization with coronary angiography, and extracorporeal circulation.

Case Example #5

The following case is for a gastric bypass (gastroenterostomy), which is coded to 44.39 in ICD-9-CM. The code descriptor for 44.39 is Other gastroenterostomy and is categorized under category 44.3, Gastro-enterostomy without gastrectomy. In ICD-9-CM, codes are also available for percutaneous endoscopic gastrojejunostomy (44.32) and laparoscopic gastroenterostomy (44.38).

Case Description: The patient is a 33-year-old woman who is admitted for bariatric surgery for morbid obesity. The patient, who has been obese since childhood, currently weighs 150 lbs over her ideal body weight. The patient's BMI is 48.4. In the past 15 years, she has been treated for essential hypertension, hyperlipidemia, sleep apnea, chole-lithiasis, insulin resistance, oligomenorrhea, and osteoarthritis of the back, hips, and knees. She has had repeated failures of other therapeutic approaches to losing weight and has been cleared by a psychiatrist who could find no psychopathology that would make her ineligible for this procedure. Her group health insurance has approved payment for the surgery. The patient underwent an open gastric bypass with Roux-en-Y limb to jejunum (gastroenterostomy) procedure, had an uneventful postoperative recovery in the hospital, and was discharged for follow-up in the office. During this hospital stay, hypertension, hyperlipidemia, insulin resistance, and osteoarthritis of the spine and multiple joints were also treated.

Case Explanation: The gastric bypass (gastroenterostomy) would code to the root operation Bypass (0D160ZA) in ICD-10-PCS. When coding this procedure, one would need to carefully review the operative report because there may be various ways that this procedure is actually performed. In this limited scenario, the procedure code is based on this limited documentation. Bypass procedures are coded by identifying the body part bypassed "from" (stomach with the fourth character of 6) and the body part bypassed "to" (jejunum with the seventh character of A).

A Roux-en-Y anastomosis is defined as a Y-shaped anastomosis in which the small intestine is included; after division of the small intestine segment, the distal end is implanted into another organ, such as the stomach or esophagus, and the proximal end into the small intestine below the anastomosis (Dorland 2003).

Case Example #6

This cholangiography will be presented in chapter 12 in the Ancillary section. Only address the cholecystojejunostomy here.

The following case is for the Roux-en-Y cholecystojejunostomy, which is coded to 51.32 in ICD-9-CM. The code descriptor for 51.32 is Anastomosis of gallbladder to intestine and is categorized under category 51.3, Anastomosis of gallbladder or bile duct

Case Description: A 3-month-old infant is born with a biliary atresia. The patient has severe obstructive jaundice due to the congenital condition. The patient was admitted and the diagnosis is confirmed by surgical exploration with operative cholangiography. The biliary atresia is treated with laparoscopic Roux-en-Y cholecystojejunostomy of the gallbladder.

Case Explanation: To code the Roux-en-Y cholecystojejunostomy procedure, the root operation is bypass, with the body system of hepatobiliary system and pancreas (0F144ZB). A cholecystojejunostomy is an anastomosis of the gallbladder and the jejunum. In ICD-10-PCS, the code for the body part (gallbladder) (character 4) is the origin of the bypass, and the qualifier (character 7) (jejunum) identifies the destination of the bypass.

Chapter 8

Medical and Surgical Section: Root Operations That Include Other Repairs and Root Operations Involving Examination Only

Root Operations That Include Other Repairs

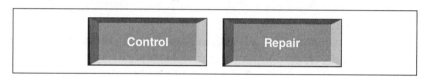

Control: 3

Definition   Stopping, or attempting to stop, postprocedural bleeding

Explanation The site of the bleeding is coded as an anatomical region and not to a specific body part

Examples   Control of post-prostatectomy hemorrhage, control of post-tonsillectomy hemorrhage

Control is used to represent a small range of procedures performed to treat postprocedural bleeding. If performing Bypass, Detachment, Excision, Extraction, Reposition, Replacement, or Resection is required to stop the bleeding, then Control is not coded separately.

Coding Guideline: B3.7 Control vs. More Definitive Root Operations

The root operation Control is defined as, "Stopping, or attempting to stop, postprocedural bleeding." If an attempt to stop postprocedural bleeding is initially unsuccessful, and to stop the bleeding requires performing any of the definitive root operations Bypass, Detachment,

Excision, Extraction, Reposition, Replacement, or Resection, then that root operation is coded instead of Control.

Example: Resection of spleen to stop postprocedural bleeding is coded to Resection instead of Control.

Note: Control includes irrigation or evacuation of hematoma done at the operative site. Both irrigation and evacuation may be necessary to clear the operative field and effectively stop the bleeding and are considered part of the procedure.

Additional Examples of Control Procedures

- Reopening laparotomy site with ligation of arterial bleeder
- Hysteroscopy with cautery of post-hysterectomy oozing and evacuation of clot (this is Control and not Destruction because the intent is to stop postoperative bleeding)
- Exploration and ligation post-op arterial bleeder, forearm
- Control post-operative retroperitoneal bleeding via laparotomy
- Reopening thoracotomy site with drainage and control of post-op hemopericardium
- Arthroscopy with drainage of hemarthrosis at previous operative site of knee

Repair: Q

Definition   Restoring, to the extent possible, a body part to its normal anatomic structure and function

Explanation   Used only when the method to accomplish the repair is not one of the other root operations

Examples   Herniorrhaphy, suture of laceration

The root operation Repair represents a broad range of procedures for restoring the anatomic structure of a body part such as suture of lacerations. Repair also functions as the "not elsewhere classified (NEC)" root operation, to be used when the procedure performed does not meet the definition of one of the other root operations. Fixation devices are included for procedures to repair the bones and joints.

Limited NEC Code Options

ICD-9-CM often designates codes as "not elsewhere classified" (NEC) or "other specified" versions of a procedure throughout the code set. NEC options are also provided in ICD-10-PCS, but only for specific, limited use.

In the Medical and Surgical section, the two significant NEC options are:

- Root operations value Q, Repair
- Device value Y, Other Device.

The root operation Repair is a true NEC value. It is used only when the procedure performed is not one of the other root operations in the Medical and Surgical section.

Additional Examples of Repair Procedures

- Inguinal herniorrhaphy (herniorrhaphy with Marlex mesh is coded to Supplement, not Repair)
- Suture radial nerve laceration
- Laparotomy with suture blunt force duodenal laceration
- Perineoplasty with repair of old obstetric laceration
- Suture right biceps tendon laceration
- Closure abdominal wall stab wound

Apply Knowledge to Transition from Coding in ICD-9-CM to ICD-10-PCS

Case Example #1

The following case is for the control of post-op bleeding in a patient recently having a heart valve replaced. This is coded to 39.41 in ICD-9-CM. The code descriptor for 39.41 is Control of hemorrhage following vascular surgery and is categorized under category 39.4, Revision of vascular procedure.

Case Description: The patient had mitral valve replacement. After surgery, there was a drop in hemoglobin and the patient was taken back to surgery for a reopening of the thoracotomy site with drainage and control of the post-op hemopericardium.

Case Explanation: The control of the post-op bleeding procedure would code to the root operation Control (0W3C0ZZ) in ICD-10-PCS. Control includes irrigation or evacuation of a hematoma done at the operative site. Because there is documentation of drainage at the site, drainage would not be the root operation because the intent of the procedure is to control the post-op bleeding. Under control, documentation states that if a bypass, detachment, excision, extraction, reposition, replacement, or resection was required to stop the bleeding, then those root operations would be coded rather than control. In other situations however, control is the root operation selected.

Case Example #2

The following case is for the control of a bleeding duodenal ulcer. This is coded to 44.43 in ICD-9-CM. The code descriptor for 44.43 is Endoscopic control of gastric or duodenal bleeding and is categorized under category 44.4, Control of hemorrhage and suture of ulcer of stomach or duodenum.

Case Description: The patient was a 55-year-old man who was admitted to the hospital by his private physician after vomiting bright red blood during a visit in the office the same day. A consultation with a gastroenterologist was requested. After radiological studies, it was determined that the patient had an acute duodenal ulcer that was hemorrhaging. The patient consented to an upper gastrointestinal endoscopy. During the esophagogastroduodenoscopy, the physician located several bleeding points in the duodenum and proceeded to control the bleeding through the endoscope with thermocoagulation to the vessel with a heater probe. It was also noted that the patient had a sliding hiatal hernia. The patient recovered from the procedure well, suffered no further episodes of vomiting or bleeding, and was discharged with medications. Follow-up appointments with his physicians were scheduled.

Case Explanation: At first glance, this procedure might be thought to be a control root operation. This is where the understanding and correct interpretation of the root operation definitions is critical. Control is defined as stopping, or attempting to stop, postprocedural bleeding. This is not the case in this example. The patient presented with a spontaneous bleeding ulcer. In this case the patient had an inspection (upper gastrointestinal endoscopy) but during that inspection, the bleeding was stopped

with thermocoagulation with a heater probe. This best fits the definition of the root operation Destruction (0D598ZZ) in ICD-10-PCS. The
inspection is not separately coded because inspection performed in order
to achieve the objective of a procedure is not coded separately.

Case Example #3

The following case is for the repair of a right inguinal hernia, which is
coded to 53.01 in ICD-9-CM. The code descriptor for 53.01 is Other
and open repair of direct inguinal hernia and is categorized under
category 53.0, Other unilateral repair of inguinal hernia. Code 53.01
includes direct and indirect hernias.

Case Description:

History: This is a 28-year-old man with a recurrent, reducible right
inguinal hernia noted on examination. He had undergone surgical
repair of a right inguinal hernia 2 years ago, so he was familiar with
the symptoms and called this surgeon's office for an appointment. The
young man works in a construction job building scaffolds and, therefore, does heavy lifting on a daily basis. Otherwise, he is healthy, well-
nourished, and well-built with no other surgical history and no other
evident medical problems. Preoperative testing, including a chest x-ray,
EKG, and usual laboratory work, were all within normal limits. He is
admitted to the hospital for this procedure, as it is a recurrent hernia,
and the procedure will require that he have highly limited mobility
for the next 36–48 hours. He will also stay in the hospital for a short
recovery period. He will then be placed on work-related disability and
advised to avoid working for a minimum of 4 weeks.

Operative Findings: A recurrent, reducible right inguinal hernia, direct
and indirect, was found. There was no strangulation or gangrene. A right
inguinal hernia repair (Bassini) with high ligation was performed.

Procedure: The patient was taken to the operating room and placed in
a supine position on the table. After satisfactory general anesthesia was
administered, the right groin was prepped with Betadine scrub and paint
and draped in the usual sterile fashion. The skin overlying the groin was
incised through the external inguinal ring exposing the spermatic cord.
The cord was then mobilized and a Penrose drain passed around it at
the level of the pubic tubercle. The cord was skeletonized proximally,

revealing a very small indirect inguinal hernia sac. The sac was dissected away from the remainder of the cord structure which was left free of injury. The sac was opened and found to contain no contents. There was also a direct inguinal hernia noted but no femoral hernia noted. The sac was twisted and ligated with 3-0 silk suture ligature. The remainder of the sac was amputated. A floor repair was performed as described by Bassini with interrupted 0 Ethibond sutures between the transversalis fascia and the shelving edge of the inguinal ligament. The internal inguinal ring was left to the size of the tip of an adult finger and the initial suture medially was from the transversalis fascia into the aponeurosis over the pubic tubercle. Upon completion, hemostasis was adequate and no relaxing incision was necessary. Spermatic cord was returned to the inguinal canal. The ilioinguinal nerve was blocked prior to this procedure and reblocked again with 0.5% Marcaine and epinephrine solution. The pubic tubercle, inguinal ligament and subcutaneous tissue were also anesthetized with 0.5% Marcaine and epinephrine solution. The external oblique was then closed with running 3-0 Vicryl. The wound was copiously irrigated and the skin closed with skin clips. A sterile dressing was applied. Gentle traction was placed on the right testicle to fully return it to the scrotum. The patient was transferred to the recovery room in stable condition.

Case Explanation: The repair of an inguinal hernia (without mesh) would code to the root operation Repair (0YQ50ZZ) in ICD-10-PCS. In ICD-10-PCS, there is no mention of the diagnosis in the procedure coding, so the code assigned does not specify if the hernia is direct or indirect. The laterality is specified however, as is the approach. In this procedure, there is documentation that the approach was open, rather than percutaneous or percutaneous endoscopic.

Case Example #4

The following case is for the repair of the vagina (cystocele), which is coded to 70.51 in ICD-9-CM. The code descriptor for 70.51 is Repair of cystocele and is categorized under category 70.5, Repair of cystocele and rectocele. This code is Indexed under repair, cystocele.

Case Description: A 52-year-old woman was admitted to the hospital with urinary stress incontinence and is scheduled for surgical repair of a paravaginal cystocele. An open anterior colporrhaphy is performed to repair the cystocele that was causing the incontinence. The patient has mild type 2 diabetes that is also treated during the hospital stay.

Case Explanation: A vaginal repair procedure would code to the root operation Repair (0U**Q**G0ZZ) in ICD-10-PCS. During the colporrhaphy, a surgical repair of a defect in the vaginal wall is performed. The defect can be a cystocele (bladder protrudes into the vagina) or a rectocele (rectum protrudes into the vagina).

In ICD-9-CM, the procedure is linked to a diagnosis (cystocele) but this is not the case in ICD-10-PCS.

Case Example #5

The following case is for the repair of a rotator cuff, which is coded to 83.63 in ICD-9-CM. The code descriptor for 83.63 is Rotator cuff repair and is categorized under category 83.6, Suture of muscle, tendon, and fascia.

Case Description: The patient, a 48-year-old female, was admitted to the hospital for surgical repair of a massive rotator cuff tear of the tendon in her right shoulder. The patient was known to have hypertension, but it was well controlled and she received medical clearance for surgery. The patient has had pain, weakness, and limited range of motion in her right shoulder, which has been present for several years and has been getting progressively worse. Several years ago she had a fall and injured her right hip but doesn't remember her shoulder being injured at that time. The patient was taken to surgery and placed under general anesthesia. The surgeon found a complete tear of the rotator cuff that appeared nontraumatic, and significant tenosynovitis of the shoulder. The surgeon performed a rotator cuff repair in an open approach because of the size of the rotator cuff tear. The patient was kept overnight in the hospital, received her anti-hypertensive medication, and was discharged to home on day 2 with a follow-up appointment with the surgeon in 10 days.

Case Explanation: A tendon repair would code to the root operation Repair (0L**Q**10ZZ) in ICD-10-PCS. The laterality can be specified in ICD-10-PCS. The rotator cuff is comprised of a group of four muscles: supraspinatus, infraspinatus, teres minor, and subscapularis muscles. The tendons at the ends of these muscles can become torn, causing restricted movement of the arm.

Case Example #6

The following case is for the suture of a laceration, which is coded to 86.59. The code descriptor for 86.59 is Closure of skin and subcutaneous tissue of other sites and is categorized under category 86.5, Suture or other closure of skin and subcutaneous tissue.

Case Description: The patient, a 22-year-old man, was brought to the emergency department by friends after being involved in a fight. Multiple lacerations were noted on both hands. One laceration in particular across the metacarpal area of the right hand required suturing of the subcutaneous tissue and skin, which was done in the emergency department. The patient is discharged and is to be seen by his physician in five days for follow-up.

Case Explanation: A repair of the subcutaneous tissue would code to the root operation Repair (0J**Q**J0ZZ) in ICD-10-PCS. When coding this procedure in ICD-9-CM, there are limited options available. Some specific sites (such as eyelid, ear, and breast) are available, but most other repairs are reported with code 86.59. In ICD-10-PCS, the site can be specified—such as upper leg, lower leg, or foot—and laterality is also available. In addition, depth will guide the selection of the body system, whether it is of the skin only or involves deeper tissues such as subcutaneous tissue and fascia. The approach value is open, though the surgical exposure may have been created by the wound itself.

Root Operations Involving Examination Only

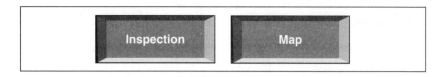

Inspection: J

Definition	Visually and/or manually exploring a body part
Explanation	Visual exploration may be performed with or without optical instrumentation. Manual exploration may be performed directly or through intervening body layers
Examples	Diagnostic arthroscopy, exploratory laparotomy

The root operation Inspection represents procedures where the sole objective is to examine a body part. Procedures that are discontinued without any other root operation being performed are also coded to Inspection.

Coding Guideline: B3.11a. Inspection Procedures

Inspection of a body part(s) performed in order to achieve the objective of a procedure is not coded separately.

> **Example:** Fiberoptic bronchoscopy performed for irrigation of bronchus, only the irrigation procedure is coded.

Coding Guideline: B3.11b

If multiple tubular body parts are inspected, the most distal body part inspected is coded. If multiple non-tubular body parts in a region are inspected, the body part that specifies the entire area inspected is coded.

> **Examples:** Cystourethroscopy with inspection of bladder and ureters is coded to the ureter body part value.

Exploratory laparotomy with general inspection of abdominal contents is coded to the peritoneal cavity body part value.

Coding Guideline: B3.11c

When both an Inspection procedure and another procedure are performed on the same body part during the same episode, if the Inspection procedure is performed using a different approach than the other procedure, the Inspection procedure is coded separately.

Example: Endoscopic Inspection of the duodenum is coded separately when open Excision of the duodenum is performed during the same procedural episode.

Procedures that are discontinued without any other root operation being performed are coded to Inspection.

Additional Examples of Inspection Procedures

- Diagnostic colposcopy with examination of cervix
- Thoracotomy with exploration of right pleural cavity
- Diagnostic laryngoscopy
- Exploratory arthrotomy left knee
- Colposcopy with diagnostic hysteroscopy
- Digital rectal exam
- Endoscopy maxillary sinus
- Laparotomy with palpation of liver
- Transurethral diagnostic cystoscopy
- Colonoscopy

Map: K

Definition   Locating the route of passage of electrical impulses and/or locating functional areas in a body part

Explanation   Applicable only to the cardiac conduction mechanism and the central nervous system

Examples   Cardiac mapping, cortical mapping

Mapping represents a very narrow range of procedures. Procedures include only cardiac mapping and cortical mapping.

The only 2 Body systems under Map are the Central Nervous System (00K) and Heart and Great Vessels (02K).

Additional Examples of Map Procedures

- Percutaneous mapping of basal ganglia
- Heart catheterization with cardiac mapping
- Intraoperative whole brain mapping via craniotomy
- Mapping left cerebral hemisphere
- Intraoperative cardiac mapping during open heart surgery

Apply Knowledge to Transition from Coding in ICD-9-CM to ICD-10-PCS

Case Example #1

The following case is for an esophagogastroduodenoscopy (EGD), which is coded to 45.13 in ICD-9-CM. The code descriptor for 45.13 is Other endoscopy of small intestine and is categorized under category 45.1, Diagnostic procedures on small intestine. The EGD was performed to diagnose the GI bleeding while the patient was a hospital inpatient.

Case Description: A 75-year-old man was admitted to the hospital after coming to the emergency department after having a black melanotic stool the day before and on the day of admission. He had no pain, nausea, or vomiting but felt a little "light-headed." Testing in the emergency department found grossly guaiac positive stools. His admitting diagnosis was gastrointestinal bleeding. The patient has an extensive past medical and surgical history including:

1. Coronary artery bypass graft 7 years ago after a myocardial infarction with no symptoms today, but takes one baby aspirin a day
2. Recurrent deep vein thrombosis of lower extremity and recurrent pulmonary emboli, currently taking Coumadin to prevent recurrence
3. History of congestive heart failure currently taking Lanoxin and Dyazide
4. History of arthritis currently taking Tolectin
5. History of hyperlipidemia currently taking Lescol

6. Suspected carcinoma of the pancreas with an exploratory laparotomy 5 years ago that only proved pancreatitis to be present, no malignancy
7. Appendectomy, colon resection done years before for what sounds like a bowel obstruction and stomach surgery for what the patient calls a "blockage"
8. Large ventral hernia related to his left upper quadrant abdominal incision from past surgery that is of no consequence at this time

During this hospital stay, he was given intravenous medications, vitamin K injection, and 2 units fresh frozen plasma to reverse the effects of the Coumadin. Serial CBCs were done which showed marginally low hemoglobin and hematocrit but nothing requiring treatment for anemia. An EGD was performed by the gastroenterologist who documented a hiatal hernia with reflux esophagitis, a proximal jejunal ulcer that appeared to have been bleeding, but there is no bleeding now, and evidence of a past gastrojejunostomy. The EGD was simply diagnostic, no biopsies were taken.

Case Explanation: The EGD procedure would code to the root operation Inspection (0DJ08ZZ) in ICD-10-PCS. This is Inspection and not Excision because no tissue or biopsy was taken. In ICD-10-PCS, the inspection of the gastrointestinal system identifies the upper intestinal tract, stomach, and lower intestinal tract as body parts. The approach for an EGD is character 8: via natural or artificial opening endoscopic.

Case Example #2

The following case is for an exploratory laparotomy, which is coded to 54.11 in ICD-9-CM. The code descriptor for 54.11 is Exploratory laparotomy and is categorized under category 54.1, Laparotomy.

Case Description: The patient is an 84-year-old woman who was brought to the emergency department by her family upon the advice of the family physician. The patient said she had increasing abdominal pain, nausea, and some vomiting. This condition started 2 to 3 days ago, and the patient could not eat due to the nausea. Prior to this episode of illness, the patient had been reasonably well, receiving medications for hypertension and hypothyroidism. The patient was admitted. Overnight, the patient appeared to become more acutely ill, developed respiratory distress, and the rapid response team evaluated her and obtained her physician's order to transfer her to the ICU. Soon after, the patient required intubation and mechanical ventilation for acute respiratory failure. The patient had signs and symptoms of septicemia and sepsis, possibly with an intra-abdominal source. Blood cultures grew E. coli. She was taken to the operating room, where she underwent an exploratory laparotomy. The surgeons found acute bowel ischemia and gangrene involving 100% of the small bowel and the right colon. This was an inoperable condition, and the laparotomy site was closed. The family was advised of the patient's very poor prognosis and offered hospice care, which they accepted. The mechanical ventilation was discontinued, and the patient was extubated. She was kept as comfortable as possible overnight and expired in the early morning hours of hospital day 4. The physician's final diagnoses were acute ischemic and gangrenous intestine, acute respiratory failure, E. coli septicemia, hypertension, and hypothyroidism.

Case Explanation: The exploratory laparotomy would code to the root operation Inspection (0WJG0ZZ) in ICD-10-PCS. The Index in ICD-10-PCS under Laparotomy states: Exploratory—*see* Inspection, Cavity, Peritoneal, 0WJG. The general Body System (W) is used because the procedure is performed on an anatomical region rather than a specific body part. The body part selected is Peritoneal cavity (G) because the peritoneal cavity consists of a large membrane in the abdominal cavity that connects and supports the internal organs (consisting of the liver, spleen, and most of the gastrointestinal tract).

Case Example #3

The following case is for a colonoscopy, which is coded to 45.23 in ICD-9-CM. The code descriptor for 45.23 is Colonoscopy and is categorized under category 45.2, Diagnostic procedures on large intestine.

Case Description: A 50-year-old man is scheduled for an outpatient colonoscopy. The reason for the colonoscopy is stated as "change in bowel habits, family history of colon cancer, and possible colonic polyp." A colonoscopy is performed. At the conclusion of the colonoscopy, the physician documents the final diagnosis as (1) change in bowel habits, unexplained, (2) normal colon examination.

Case Explanation: A colonoscopy procedure would code to the Root Operation Inspection (0DJD8ZZ) in ICD-10-PCS. The Body Part for the colonoscopy is lower intestinal tract (D) in the Gastrointestinal system.

Case Example #4

The following case is for a right fiber-optic bronchoscopy, which is coded to 33.22 in ICD-9-CM. The code descriptor for 33.22 is Fiber-optic bronchoscopy and is categorized under category 33.2, Diagnostic procedures on lung and bronchus. In ICD-9-CM there is a distinction made between bronchoscopies that are fiber-optic (33.22) and other bronchoscopies (33.23).

Case Description: A patient is admitted for a bronchoscopy with a transbronchial lung biopsy to determine the etiology of a right mass found on recent x-ray and CT studies. The patient had been complaining of a cough and chest pressure over the past several weeks. The patient is taken to the outpatient endoscopy suite. Following administration of conscious sedation, the right fiber-optic bronchoscopy is performed. During the process to obtain the transbronchial biopsy, the patient experiences a prolonged episode of bradycardia, and the physician terminates the procedure before the biopsy is obtained. The procedure will be rescheduled after the cardiologist evaluates the patient.

Case Explanation: A bronchoscopy procedure would code to the root operation Inspection (0BJ08ZZ) in ICD-10-PCS. The Index in ICD-10-PCS provides the code 0BJ08ZZ for bronchoscopy. At first glance this case appeared to be an excision because the patient was admitted for a transbronchial lung biopsy. However, there was a complication, and the biopsy was not performed. Coding guideline B3.3 states that if the intended procedure is discontinued, code the procedure to the Root Operation performed. If a procedure is discontinued before any other Root Operation is performed, code the Root Operation Inspection of the Body Part or anatomical region inspected.

Case Example #5

The following case is for an atrioventricular (AV) conduction node ablation and map. The ablation is coded to 37.34 in ICD-9-CM. The code descriptor for 37.34 is Excision or destruction of other lesion or tissue of heart, other approach and is categorized under category 37.3, Pericardiectomy and excision of lesion of heart. The cardiac map is coded to 37.27, Cardiac mapping and is categorized under category 37.2, Diagnostic procedures on heart and pericardium. Any cardiac catheterization would be coded in addition. In this limited case scenario, documentation is not present.

Case Description: A patient with rapid atrial fibrillation that is resistant to medical management is referred to the electrophysiology (EP) laboratory for AV node ablation. He undergoes placement of peripherally placed catheters into the right atrial septum for mapping. The appropriate location for ablation is mapped and the designated area is ablated.

Case Explanation: A heart ablation procedure would code to the root operation Destruction (02583ZZ) and the cardiac conduction mapping would code to the Root Operation map (02K83ZZ). It is appropriate to assign both procedures. The percutaneous method was selected (3) because the procedures were performed through peripherally placed catheters. The atrioventricular node (AV node) is part of the electrical control system of the heart and is responsible for coordinating heart rate.

The National Heart, Lung, and Blood Institute (part of the National Institutes of Health) has an Index of Conditions available that provides information about various conditions and procedures. Under "Tests and Procedures" there is information about catheter ablation. By clicking on "What to Expect During" there is an animation that explains how the ablation procedure is performed.

Chapter 9

Medical and Surgical Section: Root Operations That Always Involve a Device

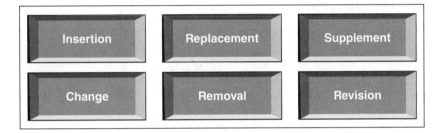

| Insertion | Replacement | Supplement |
| Change | Removal | Revision |

Insertion: H

Definition   Putting in a non-biological device that monitors, assists, performs or prevents a physiological function but does not physically take the place of a body part

Explanation   N/A

Examples   Insertion of radioactive implant, insertion of central venous catheter

The root operation Insertion represents those procedures where the sole objective is to put in a device without doing anything else to a body part. Procedures typical of those coded to Insertion include putting in a vascular catheter, a pacemaker lead, or a tissue expander.

Additional Examples of Insertion Procedures

- Port-a-cath placement
- Open placement of dual chamber pacemaker in chest wall

- Percutaneous placement of pacemaker lead into left atrium
- Percutaneous insertion of bone growth stimulator electrode, left femoral shaft
- Cystoscopy with placement of brachytherapy seeds in prostate gland
- Percutaneous placement of intrathecal infusion pump for pain management
- Percutaneous placement of Swan-Ganz catheter in superior vena cava
- Open insertion of multiple channel cochlear implant, right ear

Replacement: R

Definition Putting in or on biological or synthetic material that physically takes the place and/or function of all or a portion of a body part

Explanation The body part may have been taken out or replaced, or may be taken out, physically eradicated, or rendered nonfunctional during the Replacement procedure. A Removal procedure is coded for taking out the device used in a previous replacement procedure.

Examples Total hip replacement, bone graft, free skin graft

The objective of procedures coded to the root operation Replacement is to put in a device that takes the place of some or all of a body part. Replacement encompasses a wide range of procedures, from joint replacements to grafts of all kinds.

Note: Replacement includes taking out the body part.

Additional Examples of Replacement Procedures

- Phacoemulsification of cataract of right eye with intraocular lens implantation
- Right hip hemiarthroplasty, open
- Open aortic valve replacement using porcine valve
- Percutaneous penetrating keratoplasty of left cornea with donor matching cornea

- Excision of abdominal aorta with Gore-Tex graft replacement, open
- Open tenonectomy with graft to left ankle using cadaver graft
- Total left knee arthroplasty with insertion of total knee prosthesis
- Bilateral mastectomy with free TRAM flap reconstruction
- Right total hip replacement, open
- Partial-thickness skin graft to right lower leg, autograft

Supplement: U

Definition	Putting in or on biologic or synthetic material that physically reinforces and/or augments the function of a portion of a body part
Explanation	The biological material is non-living, or is living and from the same individual. The Body Part may have been previously replaced, and the Supplement procedure is performed to physically reinforce and/or augment the function of the replaced body part.
Examples	Herniorrhaphy using mesh, free nerve graft, mitral valve ring annuloplasty, put a new acetabular liner in a previous hip replacement

The objective of procedures coded to the root operation Supplement is to put in a device that reinforces or augments the functions of some or all of a body part. The body part may have been taken out during a previous procedure, but is not taken out as part of the Supplement procedure. Supplement includes a wide range of procedures, from hernia repairs using mesh reinforcement to heart valve annuloplasties and grafts such as nerve grafts that supplement but do not physically take the place of the existing body part.

Additional Examples of Supplement Procedures

- Open anterior colporrhaphy with polypropylene mesh
- Laparoscopic right inguinal hernia repair with Marlex mesh

- Open exchange of liner in right femoral component of previous hip replacement
- Open mitral valve annuloplasty using ring
- Percutaneous endoscopic autograft nerve graft to left radial nerve
- Implantation of CorCap cardiac support device, open
- Open abdominal wall hernia repair using synthetic mesh
- Open tendon graft using autograft
- Onlay lamellar keratoplasty of right cornea using autograft, external approach
- Open resurfacing procedure on left acetabular surface

Change: 2

Definition	Taking out or off a device from a body part and putting back an identical or similar device in or on the same body part without cutting or puncturing the skin or a mucous membrane
Explanation	All Change procedures are coded using the approach External
Examples	Urinary catheter change, gastrostomy tube change

The root operation Change represents only those procedures where a similar device is exchanged without making a new incision or puncture. Typical Change procedures include exchange of drainage devices and feeding devices.

In the root operation Change, general body part values are used when the specific body part value is not in the Table.

Additional Examples of Change Procedures

- Tracheostomy tube exchange
- Change Foley urinary catheter
- Exchange of chest tube for right pneumothorax
- Percutaneous endoscopic gastrostomy (PEG) tube exchange
- Exchange of cerebral ventriculostomy drainage tube
- Exchange of drainage tube from left hip joint

Removal: P

Definition   Taking out or off a device from a body part

Explanation   If a device is taken out and a similar device put in without cutting or puncturing the skin or mucous membrane, the procedure is coded to the root operation Change. Otherwise, the procedure for taking out a device is coded to the root operation Removal.

Examples   Drainage tube removal, cardiac pacemaker removal

Removal represents a much broader range of procedures than those for removing the devices contained in the root operation Insertion. A procedure to remove a device is coded to Removal if it is not an integral part of another root operation and regardless of the approach or the original root operation by which the device was put in.

In the root operation Removal, general body part values are used when the specific body part value is not in the table.

Additional Examples of Removal Procedures

- Removal of endotracheal tube (extubation)
- Removal of tracheostomy tube
- Removal of external fixator, left humeral head fracture
- Removal of PEG tube (non-incisional)
- Open removal of lumbar sympathetic neurostimulator
- Non-incisional removal of Swan-Ganz from superior vena cava
- Transurethral removal of brachytherapy seeds
- Incision with removal of K-wire fixation, left second metacarpal
- Cystoscopy with removal of right ureteral stent
- Removal of external fixator, left humeral fracture

Revision: W

Definition   Correcting, to the extent possible, a malfunctioning or displaced device

Explanation   Revision can include correcting a malfunctioning device by taking out and/or putting in part of the device

Examples   Adjustment of pacemaker lead, adjustment of hip
                   prosthesis

Revision is coded when the objective of the procedure is to correct the
positioning or function of a previously placed device, without taking
the entire device out and putting a whole new device in its place. A
complete re-do of the original root operation is coded to the root operation performed.

   In the root operation Revision, general body part values are used
when the specific body part value is not in the Table.

Additional Examples of Revision Procedures

- Open revision of left hip replacement, with readjustment of
  the prosthesis
- Percutaneous adjustment of position of left pacemaker lead in
  the left atrium
- Reposition of Swan-Ganz catheter in superior vena cava
- Taking out loose screw and putting larger screw in fracture
  repair plate, right fibula
- Revision of VAD reservoir placement in chest wall, open

Apply Knowledge to Transition from Coding in ICD-9-CM to ICD-10-PCS

Case Example #1

The following case is for insertion of an endotracheal tube which is
coded to 96.04 in ICD-9-CM. The code descriptor for 96.04 is Insertion
of endotracheal tube and is categorized under category 96.0, Nonoperative intubation of gastrointestinal and respiratory tracts. All endotracheal
tube insertions are coded to 96.04 as ICD-9-CM does not differentiate
the approach used to perform this procedure. The patient was subsequently placed on mechanical ventilation for 56 hours, which is coded
to 96.71, Continuous invasive mechanical ventilation for less than 96
consecutive hours. If the patient had been on the ventilator for more than
96 consecutive hours, the code would be 96.72 instead of 96.71. ICD-
9-CM also provides code 96.70 if the documentation does not indicate
the duration of the mechanical ventilation (unspecified duration).

Case Description: The patient is a 65-year-old man with stage 4 gastroesophageal junction carcinoma. He developed severe respiratory distress and was brought to the hospital emergency department and admitted. His condition progressed to acute respiratory failure, and he required intubation and mechanical ventilation for 56 hours.

Case Explanation: An intubation would code to the root operation Insertion (0BH17EZ) in ICD-10-PCS. Unlike ICD-9-CM, ICD-10-PCS does differentiate the approach used to insert the endotracheal tube which is captured with the fifth character of the code. The root operation for the mechanical ventilation is Performance (5A1945Z) which is from one of the Medical and Surgical-related sections of ICD-10-PCS. Similar to ICD-9-CM, ICD-10-PCS provides different codes depending on the number of consecutive hours the patient is on the ventilator. The fifth character, duration, captures the number of hours with the breakdown of consecutive hours being different than ICD-9-CM. In ICD-10-PCS the breakdown is less than 24 consecutive hours (3), 24-96 consecutive hours (4), and greater than 96 consecutive hours (5). However, ICD-10-PCS does not provide a code for unspecified duration of mechanical ventilation.

Case Example #2

In the following case, a percutaneous endoscopic gastrostomy (PEG) tube was placed, which is coded to 43.11 in ICD-9-CM. The code descriptor for 43.11 is Percutaneous [endoscopic] gastrostomy (PEG) which is categorized to category 43, Incision and excision of stomach. If the gastrostomy tube had been placed using another approach code 43.19, Other gastrostomy would be coded rather than 43.11.

Case Description:

Diagnosis: Residual dysphagia from previous cerebrovascular infarction and need for supplemental nutritional support

Procedure: PEG tube placement

Description of Procedure: After anesthetization of the gag reflex, the gastroscope was introduced. The abdomen had been prepped and draped as a sterile field. The light was found to transilluminate the left upper quadrant. The skin was anesthetized with 1% Xylocaine. A blunt needle was used to access the stomach percutaneously and a guide wire inserted.

The guide wire was grasped with a snare and brought through the mouth, along with the gastroscope. The feeding tube was threaded over the guide wire and brought through the abdominal wall with a small stab incision made along the guide wire. The gastroscope was reinserted and the PEG tube photo-documented. There was no evidence of bleeding or undue tension as a result of tube placement. Air was suctioned from the stomach and the gastroscope was removed. The Silastic fastener was placed on the PEG tube near the skin entrance. The PEG tube was then connected to dependent drainage. The patient tolerated the procedure well and was taken to the recovery room in satisfactory condition.

Case Explanation: The root operation for this procedure is Insertion (0D**H**64UZ) as the objective of this procedure is to insert a feeding device that assists a physiological function. Similar to ICD-9-CM, ICD-10-PCS provides distinct codes depending on the approach to performing the procedure. The fifth character of the ICD-10-PCS code captures the approach, percutaneous endoscopic (4). The sixth character captures the device, feeding device (U).

Case Example #3

Do not code the fluoroscopy in this case.

The following case is for placement of a dual chamber pacemaker which requires two codes in ICD-9-CM. The first code is 37.83 for the placement of the dual chamber pacemaker generator. The code descriptor for 37.83 is Initial insertion of dual-chamber device and is categorized under category 37, Other operations on heart and pericardium. Placement of the pacemaker generator in the subcutaneous tissue of either the chest or abdomen codes to 37.83. The second code is 37.72 for the placement of two leads, one in the right ventricle and one in the right atrium. The code descriptor for 37.72 is Initial insertion of transvenous leads (electrodes) into atrium and ventricle. ICD-9-CM also provides separate codes for placement of leads only in the ventricle (37.71) or only in the atrium (37.73).

Case Description:

Diagnosis: Symptomatic third-degree heart block

Procedure: Placement of permanent pacemaker with transvenous electrode

Description of Procedure: The patient was prepped and draped in the usual sterile fashion. The left subclavian vein was accessed and the guidewire was placed in position. A deep subcutaneous pacemaker pocket was created using the blunt dissection technique. A French-7 introducer sheath was advanced over the guidewire and the guidewire was removed. A bipolar endocardial lead model was advanced under fluoroscopic guidance and tip of pacemaker lead was positioned in the right ventricle. Next, the French-9.5 introducer sheath was advanced over a separate guidewire under fluoroscopic guidance and the guidewire was removed. Through this sheath, a bipolar atrial screw-in lead was positioned in the right atrium and the lead was screwed in. The pulse generator was then anchored in the subcutaneous pocket and the electrodes were connected to the pacemaker generator. The patient tolerated the procedure well and was taken to the recovery room in satisfactory condition.

Case Explanation: Similar to ICD-9-CM, coding this procedure in ICD-10-PCS also requires separate codes for the generator and leads. The appropriate root operation for both the placement of the generator and the leads is Insertion as follows: Insertion of generator (0JH60P2), insertion of lead into right ventricle (02HK3MA), and insertion of lead into right atrium (02H63MA). ICD-10-PCS differentiates the laterality of the chambers of the heart with the left ventricle (L) and left atrium (7) also having their own distinct body part character value. Additionally, ICD-10-PCS differentiates whether the pacemaker generator was placed in the subcutaneous tissue of the chest or abdomen.

Case Example #4

The following case is for a left total hip replacement, which is coded to 81.51 in ICD-9-CM. The code descriptor for 81.51 is Total hip replacement and is categorized under category 81, Repair and plastic operations on joint structures. Code 81.51 is used to code both right and left total hip replacement. A coding professional would assign 81.51 twice if the patient had bilateral total hip replacements. An additional code is used to identify the type of bearing surface. For this case the additional code would be 00.76 for ceramic-on-ceramic hip bearing surface.

Case Description: A 52-year-old man, a former professional athlete, was admitted to the hospital for hip replacement surgery to treat localized osteoarthritis that involved both hips. His left hip is considerably worse than his right hip. Otherwise, the patient is in good health. His past medical history included pneumonia 3 years ago and a hernia repair at age 35 years. A successful open left total hip replacement was performed using a ceramic-on-ceramic hip replacement bearing surface prosthesis. The patient was discharged 3 days later to receive physical therapy at home. He will be scheduled for the right hip replacement in 6 to 8 months.

Case Explanation: A left total hip replacement would code to the root operation Replacement (0SRB0J7) in ICD-10-PCS. The objective of this replacement procedure is to put in a synthetic device that physically takes the place and function of the patient's total left hip. The left hip replacement code includes taking out the patient's natural left hip. The fourth character of the hip replacement code differentiates whether the procedure was performed on the right (9) or left (B) hip. If the patient had a bilateral total hip replacement the coding professional would be required to apply two ICD-10-PCS codes, 0SR90J7 and 0SRB0J7. The seventh character (qualifier) captures the type of bearing surface; therefore, an additional code is not required.

Case Example #5

The following case is a phacoemulsification of cataract of the right eye with intraocular lens implantation which requires two codes in ICD-9-CM. The first code is the phacoemulsification of the cataract, which is coded to 13.41, Phacoemulsification and aspiration of cataract, and is categorized under category 13, Operations on lens. ICD-9-CM provides different extracapsular cataract extraction codes as follows: 13.2, Extracapsular extraction of lens by linear extraction technique; 13.3, Extracapsular extraction of lens by simple aspiration technique; 13.42, Mechanical phacofragmentation and aspiration of cataract by posterior route; 13.43, Mechanical phacofragmentation and other aspiration of cataract; 13.51 Extracapsular extraction of lens by temporal inferior route and 13.59, Other extracapsular extraction of lens. Additionally, ICD-9-CM differentiates an extracapsular cataract extraction versus an intracapsular cataract extraction (13.11 and 13.19). The second code is 13.71 for the insertion of intraocular lens prosthesis at the time of cataract extraction, one stage. ICD-9-CM does not differentiate laterality; therefore, the appropriate cataract extraction code would be the same whether the procedure was performed on the right or left eye.

Case Description:

Diagnosis: Cataract of the right eye

Procedure: Phacoemulsification of cataract with intraocular lens implantation, right eye

Description of Procedure: The patient was given a retrobulbar injection of 2.5 to 3.0 cc of a mixture of equal parts of 2% lidocaine with epinephrine and 0.75% Marcaine with Wydase. The patient was properly positioned on the operating table, and the area around the right eye was prepped and draped in the usual fashion. A self-retaining eyelid speculum was positioned and 4-0 silk suture passed through the tendon of the superior rectus muscle, thereby deviating the eye inferiorly. A 160 degree fornix-based conjunctival flap was created followed by a 150° corneoscleral groove with a #64 Beaver blade. A 6-0 silk suture was introduced to cross this groove at the 12 o'clock position and looped out of the operative field. An anterior capsulotomy was performed without difficulty. The corneoscleral section was opened with scissors to the left and the nucleus delivered with irrigation and gentle lens lop manipulation. Interrupted 10-0 nylon sutures were placed at both the nasal and lateral extent of the incision.

At this point, a modified C-loop posterior chamber lens was removed from its package and irrigated and inspected. It was then positioned into the inferior capsular bag without difficulty, and the superior haptic was placed behind the iris at the 12 o'clock position. The lens was rotated to a horizontal orientation. Three to four interrupted 10-0 nylon sutures were used to close the corneal sclera section. The silk sutures were removed, and the conjunctiva advanced back into its normal location and was secured with cautery burns. Approximately 20 to 30 mg of both Gentamicin and Kenalog were injected into the inferior cul-de-sac. After instillation of 2% Pilocarpine and Maxitrol ophthalmic solution, the eyelid speculum was removed and the eye dressed in a sterile fashion. The patient was taken to the recovery room in satisfactory condition.

Case Explanation: An extracapsular cataract extraction of the right eye with lens implantation would code to the root operation Replacement (08**R**J3JZ) in ICD-10-PCS. ICD-10-PCS does not differentiate extracapsular versus intracapsular technique; therefore, all cataract extractions with lens implantation of the right eye code to 08RJ3JZ.

Additionally, ICD-10-PCS does not differentiate the different types of extracapsular cataract extractions as ICD-9-CM does. The fourth character of this code differentiates whether the procedure was performed on the right eye (J) or the left eye (K).

Case Example #6

The following case is for a total revision of a right knee replacement. In ICD-9-CM this procedure would be coded to 00.80, Revision of knee replacement, total (all components) and is categorized under category 00.8, Other knee and hip procedures. ICD-9-CM also provides codes for revision of tibial component only (00.81), revision of femoral component only (00.82) and revision of patellar component only (00.83). If revision of two knee components is performed then the coding professional would code the appropriate two component codes (00.81–00.83). ICD-9-CM does not differentiate laterality; therefore, the code would be the same if performed on the left knee rather than the right. No additional code is needed to remove the original knee prosthesis.

Case Description: The patient is a 65-year-old man who had a total knee replacement on the right side 9 years previously. Up until 6 months ago, the patient enjoyed an active retirement, golfing on a daily basis and enjoying walks with his wife around a nearby nature reserve. The patient began to experience pain in the thigh near the knee and in the lower leg on the same side where the joint replacement had occurred. The patient returns to his orthopedic physician with these complaints and x-rays are taken. It appears the prosthetic joint is not in good position. The doctor makes the diagnosis of "aseptic loosening" of the prosthetic joint and recommends total knee revision arthroplasty. The patient consents to surgery and is admitted for the procedure. The physician finds he has to replace the femoral, tibial, and patellar components in order to take advantage of the new more durable prosthetic components that were not available when the patient originally had his knee replaced. The patient also was found to have mild gouty arthritis that was treated with medications during the hospital stay. The patient is discharged day 5 after surgery to receive physical therapy at home.

Case Explanation: A total revision of a right knee replacement would code to the root operation Replacement (0S**R**C0JZ) in ICD-10-PCS. The objective of this Replacement procedure was to put in a synthetic material that physically takes the place and function of the previously placed prosthesis. Similar to ICD-9-CM, ICD-10-PCS differentiates a total revision (Replacement) versus revision of only some of the knee components (Revision). In ICD-10-PCS the components of the knee being replaced are captured by the fourth character, body part, of the code. The fourth character of the code also differentiates the laterality of the procedure. Therefore, unlike ICD-9-CM, ICD-10-PCS captures whether the procedure was performed on the left versus the right knee. An additional code for Removal of the previous placed prosthesis is required in ICD-10-PCS (0S**P**C0JZ).

Case Example #7

The following case is for an open left inguinal herniorrhaphy with mesh, which is coded to 53.05 in ICD-9-CM. The code descriptor for 53.05 is Repair of inguinal hernia with graft or prosthesis, not otherwise specified and is categorized under category 53, Repair of hernia. Unilateral hernia repair codes with mesh are further subdivided according to whether the hernia is direct (53.03), indirect (53.04) or unspecified (53.05). If a unilateral hernia was repaired without mesh then a code from the range of 53.00–53.02 would be assigned. If a bilateral hernia repair were performed then the appropriate code from the range of 53.10–53.17 would be assigned. ICD-9-CM does differentiate if this procedure was performed laparoscopically rather than open. If performed laparoscopically then a code from the range of 17.11–17.13 would be assigned for a unilateral repair, and a code from the range of 17.21–17.24 would be assigned for a bilateral repair.

Case Description:

Diagnosis: Left initial inguinal hernia

Procedure: Left initial inguinal hernia repair with mesh

Description of Procedure: The patient was placed in the supine position on the OR table and general anesthesia was induced. The left groin was sterilely prepped and draped and an inguinal incision was made. This was carried down through the subcutaneous tissues until the external oblique fascia was reached. This was split in a direction parallel with its fibers, and the medial aspect of the opening included the external ring. The cord structures were encircled and the cremasteric muscle fibers divided. A piece of 3 × 5 mesh was obtained and trimmed to fit. It was placed down in the inguinal canal and tacked to the pubic tubercle. It was then run inferiorly along the pelvic shelving edge until lateral to the internal ring and tacked down superiorly using interrupted sutures of 0-Prolene. Details of the mesh were tucked underneath the external oblique fascia. The cord and nerve were allowed to drop back into the wound, and the wound was infiltrated with 30 cc of half percent Marcaine. The external oblique fascia was then closed with a running suture of 0-Vicryl. Subcutaneous tissues were approximated with interrupted sutures of 3-0 Vicryl. The skin was closed with a running subcuticular suture of 4-0 Vicryl. The patient tolerated the procedure well and was taken to the recovery room in satisfactory condition.

Case Explanation: The correct root operation for this procedure is Supplement (0YU60JZ) as the objective of this procedure is to put in synthetic material (mesh) to physically reinforce the weakened left inguinal area. Unlike ICD-9-CM, ICD-10-PCS does not differentiate whether the hernia is direct or indirect. If a unilateral hernia was repaired without mesh, then the root operation would be Repair instead of Supplement. If this repair had been performed on the right instead of left inguinal hernia, the code would be 0YU50JZ instead of 0YU60JZ. ICD-10-PCS also differentiates the type of mesh material with the sixth character, device, of the code. The device selections are autologous tissue substitute (7), synthetic substitute (J) and nonautologous tissue substitute (K). If a bilateral hernia repair was performed, the coding professional would assign two codes, one for right hernia repair and one for left hernia repair. ICD-10-PCS does not have a combination code similar to ICD-9-CM for bilateral hernia repairs. Similar to ICD-9-CM, ICD-10-PCS differentiates an open versus laparoscopic hernia repair. The different approaches are captured with the fifth character, approach, of the ICD-10-PCS code.

Case Example #8

The following case is for a posterior colporrhaphy with Gynemesh which requires two codes in ICD-9-CM. The first code is 70.55 for the colporrhaphy with Gynemesh. The code descriptor for 70.55 is Repair of rectocele with graft or prosthesis and is categorized under category 70.5, Repair of cystocele and rectocele. In the Tabular List there is an instruction note to "use additional code for biological substance (70.94) or synthetic substance (70.95), if known." In this case the substance is synthetic so the additional code of 70.95 would be coded in addition to the 70.55. Code 70.55 would be coded for the various approaches used to perform this procedure as ICD-9-CM does not differentiate according to approach. The coding professional would code 70.52 if the posterior colporrhaphy had been performed without mesh.

Case Description:

Diagnosis: Rectocele

Procedure: Posterior colporrhaphy with Gynemesh

Description of Procedure: The patient was placed on the OR table and general anesthesia was induced. An incision was made into the vaginal skin and the defect in the underlying fascia was identified. Attention was then turned to the posterior wall. Two Allis clamps were placed at the mucocutaneous junction in the region of the fourchette, and another clamp was placed at the apex of the rectocele.

The tissue between the distal clamps and the fourchette was excised, and carefully measured so that the introitus would be a 3-finger introitus. The posterior vaginal mucosa was then incised in the midline by sharp and blunt dissection. The mucosa was then dissected to the level at the Allis clamp at the apex of the rectocele, and dissected with blunt and sharp dissection from the underlying tissue. The rectocele was then imbricated using mattress sutures of 2-0 Vicryl and the area of the levator ani reinforced with Gynemesh. Two sutures of 2-0 Vicryl were taken in the elevator ani muscle, the excess posterior vaginal mucosa excised, and then closed with interrupted sutures of 2-0 Vicryl. The perineal muscles were then approximated in the midline in layers, using 2-0 Vicryl, after which the perineal skin was approximately using interrupted sutures of 2-0 Vicryl. The speculum was removed and the patient was taken to the recovery room in satisfactory condition.

Case Explanation: An open posterior colporrhaphy with Gynemesh would code to the root operation Supplement (0UUG0JZ) in ICD-10-PCS. Only one code is required for this procedure in ICD-10-PCS as the sixth character captures whether the device was an autologous tissue substitute (7), synthetic substitute (J), or a nonautologous tissue substitute (K). ICD-10-PCS does capture the approach with the fifth character of the code. If this procedure had been performed without mesh then Repair not Supplement would be the correct root operation.

Case Example #9

The following case is for a replacement of a tracheostomy tube which is coded to 97.23 in ICD-9-CM. The code descriptor for 97.23 is Replacement of tracheostomy tube and is categorized under category 97, Replacement and removal of therapeutic appliances.

Case Description: The patient was admitted for pneumonia. The patient is also ventilator dependent and has a tracheostomy tube in place. During this admission it was necessary to replace the tracheostomy tube. This procedure was performed by exchanging the old tracheostomy tube with a similar tube. It was not necessary to make a new incision during the exchange of tracheostomy tubes.

Case Explanation: The correct root operation for this procedure is Change (0B21XFZ) as the objective of this procedure is to exchange a similar device (tracheostomy tube) without making a new incision or puncture. All change procedures are coded using the approach External (X) in ICD-10-PCS.

Case Example #10

The following case is a removal of an external fixator from the left radius which is coded to 78.63 in ICD-9-CM. The code descriptor for 78.63 is Removal of implanted devices from radius and ulna and is categorized to category 78, Other operations on bones, except facial bones. Of note is that code 78.63 is coded for various different types of implanted devices in a bone. For example, in addition to the removal of an external fixator device, this code is also used for removal of internal fixation devices, bone growth stimulators, intramedullary fixation devices, and any type of synthetic substitute. Additionally, this code is used for the various approaches to perform the procedure, as ICD-9-CM does not differentiate this procedure by the type of approach. Also of note is that this code is used to code the removal of an implanted device in the right radius, the left radius, the right ulna and/or the left ulna.

Case Description:

Procedure: Removal of external fixation device from left radius

Description of Procedure: The patient was taken to the operating room and general anesthesia was induced. The left upper extremity was prepped and draped in a sterile fashion. A tourniquet was placed at

225 mm of pressure. The external fixator was percutaneously removed using the appropriate wrench. The four pins in the left radius were then removed manually, as well as with the drill. The wounds were irrigated with antibiotic solution and a sterile dressing applied. The patient was then taken to the recovery room in satisfactory condition.

Case Explanation: The removal of an external fixation device from the left radius would code to the root operation Removal (0PPJ35Z) in ICD-10-PCS. The sixth character of the ICD-10-PCS code does capture the specific device being removed from the left radius as follows: internal fixation device (4), external fixation device (5), autologous tissue substitute (7), synthetic substitute (J), nonautologous tissue substitute (K), drainage device (0) or bone growth stimulator (M). Additionally, the fifth character of the code indicates the approach used to perform the procedure. Also of note is that the fourth character of the code differentiates radius versus ulna, including laterality.

Case Example #11

The following is a case for removal of a sacral nerve stimulator which requires two codes in ICD-9-CM. The first code is 04.93 with the code descriptor being Removal of peripheral neurostimulator lead(s) and is categorized under category 04.9, Other operations on cranial and peripheral nerves. A note appears in the Tabular List under 04.93 instructing the coding professional to "code also any removal of neurostimulator pulse generator (86.05)". ICD-9-CM does not have a specific code for removal of a sacral nerve neurostimulator lead(s). Instead, code 04.93 is used to remove the leads of a neurostimulator for any peripheral nerve or cranial nerve and also for leads in stomach and/or anus. Additionally this code is used for all approaches to remove the lead(s). The code descriptor for 86.05 is Incision with removal of foreign body or device from skin and subcutaneous tissue and is categorized under category 86.0, Incision of skin and subcutaneous tissue. Code 86.05 is used for the removal of any type of device in either the skin or subcutaneous tissue. For example, in addition to using this code for removal of the neurostimulator generator, code 86.05 is also used to remove tissue expanders, vascular access devices, contraceptive devices, drainage devices, and infusion pumps. This code is also used for the removal of a foreign body with incision. Additionally, this code is not specific to the subcutaneous tissue and fascia of a particular body area and is used for removal of a device from areas such as the anterior or posterior neck, chest, back, abdomen, perineum, right or left upper arm, and right or left lower leg. Lastly, ICD-9-CM does not differentiate the approach used to perform this procedure; therefore code 86.05 is used for any approach when performing this procedure.

Case Description:

Diagnosis: Neurogenic bladder with an implanted sacral nerve stimulator

Procedure: Removal of InterStim sacral nerve stimulator

Description of Procedure: The patient was brought to the operating room, given a light intravenous anesthetic and laid in the prone position. The area overlying the InterStim neurostimulator was infiltrated using 1% lidocaine mixed with 0.35% Marcaine. Once this was done, an incision was made over this and dissection was carried down to the InterStim neurostimulator. The device was removed from its pouch. The leads, which were tunneled down to the S3 foramina, were identified and with careful manipulation we were able to remove in their entirety. Once this was done, hemostasis was obtained. The wound was copiously irrigated using antibiotic solution. The 3-0 Vicryl pop-offs were used to close the subcutaneous tissue, 4-0 Monocryl was used to close the skin. The patient tolerated the procedure well and was taken to the recovery room in stable condition.

Case Explanation: Similar to ICD-9-CM, a removal of a sacral nerve stimulator requires two codes in ICD-10-PCS. The two procedures performed were the removal of the neurostimulator lead(s) and the removal of the neurostimulator generator. The root operation for the removal of the lead(s) is Removal (01**P**Y0MZ) as the objective of this procedure was to take out the neurostimulator lead(s) from the sacral nerve. In ICD-10-PCS code 01PY0MZ is used to remove a neurostimulator lead(s) from any peripheral nerve. The fifth character of this code captures the approach used to perform the procedure. The sixth character of the code specifies the type of device removed, with character value M being specifically for neurostimulator leads. The root operation for the removal of the neurostimulator generator is also Removal (0J**P**T0MZ) in ICD-10-PCS. Code 0JPT0MZ is used to remove a neurostimulator generator from the subcutaneous tissue and fascia anywhere in the trunk region.

Case Example #12

The following case is for an adjustment of a dislodged lead in the right ventricle, which is coded to 37.75 in ICD-9-CM. The code descriptor for 37.75 is Revision of lead (electrodes) and is categorized under category 37, Other operations on heart and pericardium. This code is used to revise leads for various types of pacemakers and defibrillators. Additionally, ICD-9-CM does not provide distinct codes for the various approaches used to perform this procedure.

Case Description: The patient is a 74-year-old male who had a dual chamber pacemaker inserted 2 months ago for sick sinus syndrome. The lead in the right ventricle has become dislodged and the patient will need to undergo an adjustment of this lead. The patient was taken to the operating room where a percutaneous adjustment of the lead in the right ventricle was performed without incidence.

Case Explanation: The correct root operation for this procedure is Revision (02WA3MZ), as the objective of this procedure is to correct, to the extent possible, the dislodged or displaced lead. Similar to ICD-9-CM, code 02WA3MZ is used for the revision of any cardiac lead. ICD-10-PCS does provide distinct codes for the various approaches used to perform this procedure. The approach is captured with the fifth character.

Chapter 10

Medical and Surgical Section: Root Operations That Include Other Objectives

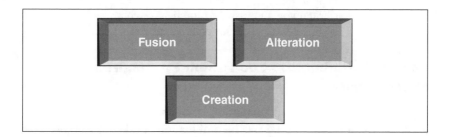

Fusion: G

Definition	Joining together portions of an articular body part rendering the articular body part immobile
Explanation	The body part is joined together by fixation device, bone graft, or other means
Examples	Spinal fusion, ankle arthrodesis

A limited range of procedures is represented in the root operation Fusion, because fusion procedures are by definition only performed on the joints. Qualifier values are used to specify whether a vertebral joint fusion uses an anterior or posterior approach, and whether the anterior or posterior column of the spine is fused.

Coding Guideline: B3.10a Fusion Procedures of the Spine

The body part coded for a spinal vertebral joint(s) rendered immobile by a spinal fusion procedure is classified by the level of the spine (for

example, thoracic). There are distinct body part values for a single vertebral joint and for multiple joints at each spinal level.

> **Example:** Body part values specify Lumbar Vertebral Joint, Lumbar
> Vertebral Joints, 2 or More and Lumbosacral Vertebral Joint.

Coding Guideline: B3.10b Fusion Procedures of the Spine

If multiple vertebral joints are fused, a separate procedure is coded for
each vertebral joint that uses a different device and/or qualifier.

> **Example:** Fusion of lumbar vertebral joint, posterior approach, ante-
> rior column and fusion of lumbar vertebral joint, posterior
> approach, and posterior column are coded separately.

Coding Guideline: B3.10c Fusion Procedures of the Spine

Combinations of devices and materials are often used on a vertebral joint
to render the joint immobile. When combinations of devices are used on
the same vertebral joint, the device value coded for the procedure is as
follows: If an interbody fusion device is used to render the joint immobile (alone or containing other material like bone graft), the procedure
is coded with the device value Interbody Fusions Device; if internal
fixation is used to render the joint immobile and an interbody fusion
device is *not* used, the procedure is coded with the device value Internal
Fixation Device; if bone graft is the *only* device used to render the joint
immobile, the procedure is coded with the device value Nonautologous
Tissue Substitute or Autologous Tissue Substitute, and if a mixture of
autologous and nonautologous bone graft (with or without biological or
synthetic extenders or binders) is used to render the joint immobile, code
the procedure with the device value Autologous Tissue Substitute.

> **Examples:** Fusion of a vertebral joint using a cage style interbody
> fusion device containing morselized bone graft is coded to
> the device Interbody Fusion Device.
>
> Fusion of a vertebral joint using a bone dowel interbody
> fusion device made of cadaver bone and packed with a
> mixture of local morselized bone and demineralized bone
> matrix is coded to the device Interbody Fusion Device.

Fusion of a vertebral joint using rigid plates affixed with screws and reinforced with bone cement is coded to the device Internal Fixation Device.

Fusion of a vertebral joint using both autologous bone graft and bone bank bone graft is coded to the device Autologous Tissue substitute.

Additional Examples of Fusion Procedures

- Posterior spinal fusion of the posterior column at L2–L4 levels with BAK cage interbody fusion device, open
- Interphalangeal fusion of right great toe, percutaneous pin fixation
- Arthrodesis of the right ankle, open
- Intercarpal fusion of left hand with bone bank bone graft, open
- Radiocarpal fusion of right hand with internal fixation, open
- Sacrococcygeal fusion with synthetic substitute, open

Alteration: 0

Definition   Modifying the natural anatomic structure of a body part without affecting the function of the body part

Explanation Principal purpose is to improve appearance

Examples   Face lift, breast augmentation

Alteration is coded for all procedures performed solely to improve appearance. All methods, approaches, and devices used for the objective of improving appearance are coded here.

Because some surgical procedures can be performed for either medical or cosmetic purposes, coding for Alteration requires diagnostic confirmation that the surgery is in fact performed to improve appearance. If the procedure is done for medical conditions, then the appropriate root operation is assigned such as Extraction, Reposition, Resection, Repair, Replacement, and the others.

Additional Examples of Alteration Procedures

- Open abdominoplasty (tummy tuck)
- Bilateral breast augmentation with silicone implants, open

- Abdominal liposuction for cosmetic reasons
- Cosmetic face lift, open
- Cosmetic rhinoplasty with septal reduction and tip elevation, using local tissue graft, open
- Open cosmetic blepharoplasty of right and left lower eyelids

Creation: 4

Definition   Making a new genital structure that does not physically take the place of a body part

Explanation   Used only for sex change operations

Examples   Creation of vagina in a male, creation of penis in a female

Creation is used to represent a very narrow range of procedures. Only the procedures performed for sex change operations are included here.

If a separate procedure is performed to harvest autograft tissue, it is coded to the appropriate root operation in addition to the primary procedure.

Additional Examples of Creation Procedures

- Creation of penis in female patient using synthetic material
- Creation of vagina in male patient using tissue bank donor graft

Apply Knowledge to Transition from Coding in ICD-9-CM to ICD-10-PCS

Case Example #1

The following case is for a posterior lumbar interbody fusion of L2–L4 which requires the assignment of three procedure codes in ICD-9-CM. The first of these three codes is 81.08, Lumbar and lumbosacral fusion, posterior technique. This code identifies the level of the spine being fused in addition to the technique (anterior, lateral transverse, or posterior) used to approach the spine. ICD-9-CM does not differentiate the surgical approach (open versus percutaneous) used to perform this procedure with 81.08 being coded for all different types of approaches. The second code is 81.62, Fusion or refusion of 2–3 vertebrae. Code 81.62 indicates the number of vertebrae fused during the procedure. The final code, 84.51, Insertion of interbody spinal fusion device, identifies the device inserted. ICD-9-CM provides different codes depending on the device(s) used to fuse the spine. ICD-9-CM does not differentiate whether the posterior or anterior column of the spine was fused. Additionally, if autologous bone graft material were also used during this procedure a fourth code would be required to identify the excision of the bone graft material.

Case Description: A 57-year-old male was admitted for a spinal fusion. The patient has had severe degenerative disc disease of his lumbar spine for quite a few years. Conservative treatment for the degenerative disc disease has provided little to no relief for the patient and he has elected to have the spinal fusion. The patient was taken to the operating room where an open posterior lumbar interbody fusion (BAK cage) of the posterior column at L2–4 levels was performed without incidence. The patient was discharged from the hospital three days later.

Case Explanation: A posterior lumbar interbody fusion at L2–L4 levels would code to the root operation Fusion (0S**G**1031) in ICD-10-PCS. Only one code is required in ICD-10-PCS in comparison to the three codes in ICD-9-CM. The fourth character of the ICD-10-PCS code captures the number of vertebrae fused, and the sixth character captures the device(s) used. Additionally, ICD-10-PCS provides different codes for the approach (open versus percutaneous), which is captured with the fifth character. In the seventh character of the code, ICD-10-PCS identifies whether the posterior or anterior column of the spine was fused. This procedure involves removing the intervertebral disk(s) and then implanting a spacer or "cage" between two adjoining vertebra. In a posterior lumbar interbody fusion the cage is inserted from the back of the spine.

Case Example #2

The following case is a triple arthrodesis of the right tarsus which is coded to 81.12 in ICD-9-CM. The code descriptor for 81.12 is Triple arthrodesis and is categorized under category 81, Repair and plastic operations on joint structures. A coding professional would assign

81.12 for the various different approaches used to perform the procedure. ICD-9-CM does not differentiate whether the triple arthrodesis was performed via an open, percutaneous, or percutaneous endoscopic approach. Additionally, ICD-9-CM does not differentiate the type of device used for fusion with code 81.12 being used for all types of devices. An additional code of 77.77 is also coded for the autologous bone graft material from the left tibia.

Case Description: The patient is a 35-year-old male who is being admitted for a triple arthrodesis of the right tarsal joint due to disabling degenerative joint disease. The patient was taken to the operating room where an open triple arthrodesis of the right tarsus was performed. Metal rods in addition to autologous bone graft material from the left tibia were used for the arthrodesis. The patient tolerated the procedure well and was discharged two days later.

Case Explanation: The correct root operation for this procedure is Fusion (0S**G**H07Z) as the objective of this procedure is to join together the three joints in the hindfoot, rendering them immobile. ICD-10-PCS does allow the coder to assign separate and unique codes for each of the approaches used to perform this procedure. The different approaches are captured with the fifth character of the code. Additionally, ICD-10-PCS provides distinct codes for the various devices used to perform this procedure. The specific device is captured with the sixth character. ICD-10-PCS also allows the coding professional to differentiate whether this procedure was performed on the right or left tarsal joint. In addition to the fusion code, the coding professional would also code the excision of the graft material. A triple arthrodesis procedure consists of the surgical fusion of the talocalcaneal, talonavicular, and calcaneocuboid joints in the hindfoot.

Case Example #3

The following case is for a bilateral breast augmentation with silicone implants, which is coded to 85.54 in ICD-9-CM. The code descriptor for 85.54 is Bilateral breast implant and is categorized under category 85, Operations on the breast. Code 85.54 is used for the various approaches to perform this procedure. If the procedure had been performed unilaterally, the code 85.53 would be assigned for both the right or left breast.

Case Description: The patient is a 44-year-old female who recently lost more than 85 pounds on a weight reduction program. The patient now desires breast augmentation surgery to restore the breast volume lost as a result of the weight reduction. The patient was taken to the operating room and underwent an open bilateral breast augmentation with silicone implants. The patient tolerated the procedure well.

Case Explanation: A coding professional would use the root operation Alteration (0H0V0JZ) to code this procedure in ICD-10-PCS. The root operation Alteration is used for any procedure that is performed for cosmetic reasons or to improve the patient's appearance. The fourth character of the code captures whether the procedure is performed on the left breast, on the right breast, or bilaterally. The fifth character of the code captures the specific approach used to perform the procedure.

Case Example #4

The following case is for an abdominoplasty, which is coded to 86.83 in ICD-9-CM. The code descriptor for 86.83 is Size reduction plastic operation and is categorized in category 86, Operations on the skin and subcutaneous tissue. ICD-9-CM does not provide distinct codes for size reduction surgeries when performed on different body parts. For example, size reduction surgery on the arms, thighs, buttocks, hip, leg, and abdomen all code to 86.83. Additionally, ICD-9-CM does not distinguish the approach used to perform the size reduction surgery.

Case Description:

Procedure: Abdominoplasty (tummy tuck)

Description of Procedure: The patient was taken to the operating room and prepared and draped in the usual manner. After induction of general anesthesia, an incision was made across the lower abdomen from hip bone to hip bone. A second incision was also made around the belly button. The skin and fat were then separated from the abdominal wall. Excess skin and fat were then excised. The abdominal muscles were tightened by shortening them and suturing them together. Next a small incision was made to create a new opening for the belly button and it was brought out through the opening sutured to the new skin. Drains were placed and all incisions were closed. The patient was then taken to the recovery room in satisfactory condition.

Case Explanation: The correct root operation for this procedure is Alteration (0W0F0ZZ) as the objective of an abdominoplasty is to improve the physical appearance of the patient. ICD-10-PCS does provide specific distinct procedure codes for the different size reductions surgeries with the fourth character of the code indicating the body part the procedure is performed on. Additionally, ICD-10-PCS captures the specific approach with the fifth character of the code.

Chapter 11

Medical and Surgical-Related Section

Definitions, Descriptions and Examples of Root Operations

ICD-10-PCS contains a total of nine Medical and Surgical-related sections as shown in table 11.1.

Table 11.1. The nine Medical and Surgical-related sections

Section Value	Description
Section 1	Obstetrics
Section 2	Placement
Section 3	Administration
Section 4	Measurement and Monitoring
Section 5	Extracorporeal Assistance and Performance
Section 6	Extracorporeal Therapies
Section 7	Osteopathic
Section 8	Other Procedures
Section 9	Chiropractic

Obstetrics: 1

The seven characters in the Obstetrics section are shown in figure 11.1.

Figure 11.1.   The seven characters in the Obstetrics section

Character 1	Character 2	Character 3	Character 4	Character 5	Character 6	Character 7
Section	Body System	Root Operation	Body Part	Approach	Device	Qualifier

The Obstetrics section follows the same conventions established in the Medical and Surgical section, with all seven characters retaining the same meaning.

- **Character 2 (Body System):** One single body system, **Pregnancy**
- **Character 4 (Body Part):** Three body part values
  - ○ Products of conception
  - ○ Products of conception, retained
  - ○ Products of conception, ectopic

Root Operations

There are a total of 12 root operations in the Obstetrics section; 10 of the root operations are found in other sections of ICD-10-PCS and two are unique to the Obstetrics section. The two unique root operations to the Obstetrics section are **Abortion** and **Delivery**.

1. *Abortion*
2. Change
3. *Delivery*
4. Drainage
5. Extraction
6. Insertion
7. Inspection
8. Removal
9. Repair
10. Reposition
11. Resection
12. Transplantation

Abortion: A

Definition   Artificially terminating a pregnancy

Explanation Subdivided according to whether an additional device such as a laminaria or abortifacient is used, or whether the abortion was performed by mechanical means

Examples   Transvaginal abortion using vacuum aspiration technique

Abortion is subdivided according to whether an additional device such as a laminaria or abortifacient is used, or whether the abortion was performed by mechanical means. If either a laminaria or abortifacient is used, then the approach is via natural or artificial opening. All other abortion procedures are those done by mechanical means (the products of conception are physically removed using instrumentation) and the device value is Z, no device.

Delivery: E

Definition   Assisting the passage of the products of conception from the genital canal

Explanation Applies only to manually assisted, vaginal delivery

Example   Manually-assisted delivery

Delivery applies only to manually-assisted, vaginal delivery and is defined as assisting the passage of products of conception from the genital canal. Cesarean deliveries are coded in this section to the root operation Extraction.

Qualifier

The qualifier values in the Obstetrics section are dependent upon the root operation, approach, or body system.

Examples: Methods of extraction: low forceps, vacuum, low cervical

Methods of terminating pregnancy: laminaria, abortifacient

Substances drained: amniotic fluid, fetal cerebrospinal fluid

Coding Guideline: C1 Products of Conception

Procedures performed on the products of conception are coded to the Obstetrics section. Procedures performed on the pregnant female other than the products of conception are coded to the appropriate root operation in the Medical and Surgical section.

> **Example:**   Amniocentesis is coded to the products of conception body part in the Obstetrics section. Repair of obstetric urethral laceration is coded to the urethra body part in the Medical and Surgical section.

Coding Note: Products of Conception
- Products of conception refer to all components of pregnancy, including fetus, embryo, amnion, umbilical cord, and placenta
- There is no differentiation of the products of conception based on gestational age

Coding Guideline: C2 Procedures Following Delivery or Abortion

Procedures performed following a delivery or abortion for curettage of the endometrium or evacuation of retained products of conception are all coded in the Obstetrics section, to the root operation Extraction and the body part Products of Conception, Retained. Diagnostic or therapeutic dilation and curettage performed during times other than the postpartum or post-abortion period are all coded in the Medical and Surgical section, to the root operation Extraction and the body part Endometrium.

Placement: 2

The seven characters in the Placement section are shown in figure 11.2.

Figure 11.2.   The seven characters in the Placement section

Character 1	Character 2	Character 3	Character 4	Character 5	Character 6	Character 7
Section	Body System	Root Operation	Body Region	Approach	Device	Qualifier

The Placement section follows the same conventions established in the Medical and Surgical section, with all seven characters retaining the same meaning.

- **Character 2 (body system):** Two body system values
  - ○ Anatomical Regions
  - ○ Anatomical Orifices
- **Character 4 (body part):** Two body region types
  - ○ External body regions (for example, chest wall)
  - ○ Natural orifices (for example, mouth)

Root Operations

The root operations in the Placement section include only those procedures performed without making an incision or puncture. There are a total of seven root operations in the Placement section of which two are common to other sections: Change and Removal. The five additional Root Operations unique to the Placement section are Compression, Dressing, Immobilization, Packing, and Traction.

1. Change
2. *Compression*
3. *Dressing*
4. *Immobilization*
5. *Packing*
6. Removal
7. *Traction*

Packing: 4

Definition   Putting material in a body region or orifice

Explanation Procedures performed without making an incision or puncture

Example   Placement of nasal packing

Additional Examples of Packing Procedures

- Placement of packing material, left ear
- Packing of wound, abdominal wall
- Placement of vaginal packing
- Placement of packing material, pharynx

Immobilization: 3

Definition   Limiting or preventing motion of a body region

Explanation   Procedures to fit a device, such as splints or braces apply only to the rehabilitation setting

Example   Placement of splint on left finger

The procedures to fit a device, such as splints and braces as described in F0DZ6EZ and F0DZ7EZ, apply only to the rehabilitation setting. Splints and braces placed in other inpatient settings are coded to Immobilization, Table 2W3 in the Placement section.

Additional Examples of Immobilization Procedures

- Placement of neck brace
- Placement of cast on left lower leg
- Placement of brace on right knee
- Placement of splint on left lower arm
- Placement of back brace

Compression: 1

Definition   Putting pressure on a body region

Explanation   Procedures performed without making an incision or puncture

Example   Placement of pressure dressing on abdominal wall

Additional Examples of Compression Procedures

- Placement of intermittent pneumatic compression device, covering entire right leg
- Placement of pressure dressing on chest wall
- Placement of intermittent pressure device to lower left arm
- Placement of pressure dressing, right foot

Dressing: 2

Definition   Putting material on a body region for protection

Explanation   Procedures performed without making an incision or puncture

Example   Application of sterile dressing to head wound

Additional Examples of Dressing Procedures

- Placement of sterile dressing to lower back
- Application of sterile dressing to abdominal wall wound
- Placement of sterile dressing to neck
- Application of sterile dressing to chest wall wound

Traction: 6

Definition   Exerting a pulling force on a body region in a distal direction

Explanation   Traction in this section includes only the task performed using a mechanical traction apparatus

Example   Lumbar traction using motorized split-traction table

Traction in this section includes only the task performed using a mechanical traction apparatus. Manual traction performed by a physical therapist is coded to Manual Therapy Techniques in Section F, Physical Rehabilitation and Diagnostic Audiology.

Additional Examples of Traction Procedures

- Lumbar traction using motorized split-traction device
- Mechanical traction of left lower leg
- Mechanical traction of entire right leg
- Mechanical traction of right lower arm

Devices

- Specifies the material or device in placement procedure (for example, splint, traction apparatus, pressure dressing, bandage)
- Includes casts for fractures and dislocations
- Devices in the Placement section are off the shelf and do not require any extensive design, fabrication, or fitting
- The placement of devices that require extensive design, fabrication, or fitting are coded in the Rehabilitation section of ICD-10-PCS

Administration: 3

The seven characters in the Administration section are shown in figure 11.3.

Figure 11.3.   The seven characters in the Administration section

Character 1	Character 2	Character 3	Character 4	Character 5	Character 6	Character 7
Section	Body System	Root Operation	Body System/ Region	Approach	Substance	Qualifier

- **Character 2 (Body System):** Three body system values
  - ○ Physiological Systems and Anatomical Regions
  - ○ Circulatory
  - ○ Indwelling Device
- **Character 5 (Approach)**
  - ○ Uses values defined in the Medical and Surgical section
  - ○ The approach value for intradermal, subcutaneous, and intramuscular introduction (that is, injections) is percutaneous
  - ○ If a catheter is used to introduce a substance into a site within the circulatory system, the approach value is percutaneous
- **Character 6 (Substance)**
  - ○ Substances are specified in broad categories
  - ○ Substance values depend on body part

Coding Note: Administration Section
The Administration section includes infusions, injections and transfusions, as well as other related procedures, such as irrigation and tattooing. All codes in this section define procedures where a diagnostic or therapeutic substance is given to the patient.

Root Operations

The root operations in the Administration section are classified according to the broad category of substance administered. If the substance given is a blood product or a cleansing substance, then the procedure is coded to Transfusion and Irrigation respectively. All other substances administered, such as antineoplastic substances, are coded to the root operation, Introduction.

1. Introduction
2. Irrigation
3. Transfusion

Transfusion: 2

Definition   Putting in blood or blood products

Explanation   Substance given is a blood product or a stem cell substance

Example   Transfusion of cell saver red cells into central venous line

Additional Examples of Transfusion Procedures

- Bone marrow transplant using donor marrow from identical twin, central vein infusion
- Transfusion of cell saver red cells via central venous catheter
- Transfusion of frozen plasma via peripheral artery
- Nonautologous bone marrow transplant via central venous line
- Transfusion of nonautologous antihemophilic factor via arterial central line
- Transfusion of nonautologous Factor X via arterial line
- Transfusion of platelet cells via peripheral artery

Irrigation: 1

Definition   Putting in or on a cleansing substance

Explanation   Substance given is a cleansing substance or dialysate

Example   Flushing of eye

Coding Note: Body Part Value
For the root operation Irrigation, the body part value specifies the site of the irrigation

---

Additional Examples of Irrigation Procedures

- Peritoneal dialysis via indwelling catheter
- Percutaneous irrigation of right knee joint
- Percutaneous irrigation of peritoneal cavity

Introduction: 0

Definition	Putting in or on a therapeutic, diagnostic, nutritional, physiological, or prophylactic substance except blood or blood products
Explanation	All other substances administered, such as antineoplastic substance
Example	Nerve blood injection to median nerve

Coding Note: Substance for Mixed Steroid and Local Anesthetic
When a substance of mixed steroid and local anesthetic is given for pain control it is coded to the substance value Anti-inflammatory. The anesthetic is only added to lessen the pain of the injection.

Coding Note: Body Part Value
For the root operation Introduction the body part value specifies where the procedure occurs and not necessarily the site where the substance introduced has an effect.

Additional Examples of Introduction Procedures

- Lumbar epidural injection of mixed steroid and local anesthetic for pain control
- Transvaginal artificial insemination
- Infusion of total parenteral nutrition via central venous catheter
- Transabdominal in-vitro fertilization, implantation of donor ovum
- Infusion of thrombolytic agent via central venous catheter
- Chemocal pleurodesis using injection of tetracycline
- Nerve block injection to median nerve

Measurement and Monitoring: 4

The seven characters in the Measurement and Monitoring section are shown in figure 11.4.

Figure 11.4. The seven characters in the Measurement and Monitoring section

Character 1	Character 2	Character 3	Character 4	Character 5	Character 6	Character 7
Section	Body System	Root Operation	Body System	Approach	Function/ Device	Qualifier

- **Character 2 (body system):** Single body system value, **Physiological System**
- **Character 6 (Function/Device):** Specifies physiological or physical function being tested (for example, nerve conductivity, respiratory capacity)

Root Operations

There are only two root operations in the Measurement and Monitoring section. Measurement is the first root operation and is used when the procedure determines the level of a physiological or physical function at a point in time. Monitoring is the second root operation and is used when the procedure determines the level of a physiological or physical function repetitively over a period of time.

1. Measurement
2. Monitoring

Measurement: 0

Definition Determining the level of a physiological or physical function at a point in time

Explanation A single temperature reading is considered a measurement

Example External EKG, single reading

Additional Examples of Measurement Procedures

- Cardiac stress test, single measurement
- Peripheral venous pulse, external, single measurement
- Visual mobility test, single measurement
- Olfactory acuity test, single measurement
- Electroencephalogram, single measurement
- Cystometrogram, single measurement
- EGD with biliary flow measurement

Monitoring: 1

Definition Determining the level of a physiological or physical function repetitively over a period of time

Explanation Temperature taken every half hour for eight hours is considered monitoring

Example Urinary pressure monitoring

Additional Examples of Monitoring Procedures

- Ambulatory Holter monitoring
- Transvaginal fetal heart rate monitoring over a period of 8 hours
- Pulmonary artery wedge pressure monitoring from Swan-Ganz catheter
- Urinary pressure monitoring
- Monitoring of esophageal fluid and gas pressures

Extracorporeal Assistance and Performance: 5

The seven characters in the Extracorporeal Assistance and Performance section are shown in figure 11.5.

Figure 11.5. **The seven characters in the Extracorporeal Assistance and Performance section**

Character 1	Character 2	Character 3	Character 4	Character 5	Character 6	Character 7
Section	Body System	Root Operation	Body System	Duration	Function	Qualifier

- **Character 2 (Body System):** Single body system value, **Physiological Systems**
- **Character 5 (Duration):** Specifies whether the procedure was a single occurrence, multiple occurrence, intermittent, or continuous
- **Character 6 (Function):** Specifies the physiological function assisted or performed (for example, oxygenation, ventilation)

> **Coding Note: Character 5: Duration**
> For respiratory ventilation assistance or performance, the range of con-
> secutive hours is specified (<24 hours, 24–96 hours, or >96 hours).

Root Operations

There are three unique root operations in the Extracorporeal Assistance
and Performance section: Assistance, Performance, and Restoration.
Assistance and Performance are two variations of the same kinds of
procedures, varying only in the degree of control exercised over the
physiological function. Assistance is taking over partial control of the
physiological function and Performance is taking complete control of
the physiological function. Restoration is returning a physiological
function to its original state.

1. Assistance
2. Performance
3. Restoration

Assistance: 0

Definition	Taking over a portion of a physiological function by extracorporeal means
Explanation	Procedures that support a physiological function but do not take complete control of it, such as intra-aortic balloon pump to support cardiac output and hyperbaric oxygen treatment
Example	Hyperbaric oxygenation of wound

Additional Examples of Assistance Procedures

- Intra-aortic balloon pump (IABP), continuous
- Intermittent positive pressure breathing, 15 hours
- Extracorporeal membrane oxygenation (ECMO), intermittent
- Assistance with cardiac output using pulsatile compression, continuous

Performance: 1

Definition	Completely taking over a physiological function by extracorporeal means

Explanation Procedures in which complete control is exercised over a physiological function, such as total mechanical ventilation, cardiac pacing, and cardiopulmonary bypass

Example Cardiopulmonary bypass in conjunction with CABG

Additional Examples of Performance Procedures

- Cardiopulmonary bypass
- Hemodialysis, single encounter
- Continuous mechanical ventilation, 67 hours
- Intraoperative cardiac pacing, continuous
- Extracorporeal hepatic assistance, single encounter
- Extracorporeal membrane oxygenation (ECMO), continuous

Restoration: 2

Definition Returning, or attempting to return, a physiological function to its original state by extracorporeal means

Explanation Only external cardioversion and defibrillation procedures. Failed cardioversion procedures are also included in the definition of restoration and are coded the same as successful procedures.

Example Attempted cardiac defibrillation, unsuccessful

Additional Examples of Restoration Procedures

- Atrial cardioversion
- Defibrillation
- External cardioversion
- Closed chest cardiac massage
- Carotid sinus stimulation

Extracorporeal Therapies: 6

The seven characters in the Extracorporeal Therapies section are shown in figure 11.6.

Figure 11.6.   The seven characters in the Extracorporeal Therapies section

Character 1	Character 2	Character 3	Character 4	Character 5	Character 6	Character 7
Section	Body System	Root Operation	Body System	Duration	Qualifier	Qualifier

- **Character 2 (Body System):** Single Body System, **Physiological Systems**
- **Character 5 (Duration):** Specifies whether the procedure was single occurrence, multiple occurrence, or intermittent
- **Character 6 (Qualifier):** No specific qualifier value (Z = no qualifier)
- **Character 7 (Qualifier):** Identifies various blood components separated out in pheresis procedures

Root Operations

The 10 root operations in the Extracorporeal Therapies section are shown in table 11.2.

Table 11.2.   The 10 Root Operations in the Extracorporeal Therapies section

Section Value	Description	Definition
0	Atmospheric Control	Extracorporeal control of atmospheric pressure and composition
1	Decompression	Extracorporeal elimination of undissolved gas from body fluids
2	Electromagnetic Therapy	Extracorporeal treatment by electromagnetic rays
3	Hyperthermia	Extracorporeal raising of body temperature
4	Hypothermia	Extracorporeal lowering of body temperature
5	Pheresis	Extracorporeal separation of blood products
6	Phototherapy	Extracorporeal treatment by light rays
7	Ultrasound Therapy	Extracorporeal treatment by ultrasound
8	Ultraviolet Light Therapy	Extracorporeal treatment by ultraviolet light
9	Shock Wave Therapy	Extracorporeal treatment by shock waves

Examples of Extracorporeal Therapies Procedures

- Bili-lite UV phototherapy, single treatment
- Plasmapheresis, single treatment
- Shock wave therapy for plantar fascia, series treatment
- Donor thrombocytapheresis, single treatment
- Whole body hypothermia, single treatment
- Circulatory phototherapy, series treatment
- Transcranial magnetic stimulation, series treatment

Osteopathic: 7

The seven characters in the Osteopathic section are shown in figure 11.7.

Figure 11.7. The seven characters in the Osteopathic section

Character 1	Character 2	Character 3	Character 4	Character 5	Character 6	Character 7
Section	Body System	Root Operation	Body Region	Approach	Method	Qualifier

- **Character 2 (Body System):** Single body system value, **Anatomical Regions**
- **Character 6 (Method):** Method of osteopathic treatment; these methods are not explicitly defined in ICD-10-PCS and rely on the standard definitions as used in this specialty.

Root Operation

Treatment: 0

Definition	Manual treatment to eliminate or alleviate somatic dysfunction and related disorder
Explanation	None
Example	Fascial release of abdomen, osteopathic treatment

Coding Note: Osteopathic Section
Section 7, Osteopathic, is one of the smallest sections in ICD-10-PCS. There is a single body system, Anatomic Regions, and a single root operation, Treatment

Examples of Osteopathic Procedures

- Osteopathic manipulative treatment using high-velocity, low-amplitude forces
- Osteopathic manipulative treatment using isotonic forces
- Osteopathic manipulative treatment using isometric forces
- Osteopathic manipulative treatment using indirect forces
- Articular osteopathic treatment of cervical region

Other Procedures: 8

The seven characters in the Other Procedures section are shown in figure 11.8.

Figure 11.8.   The seven characters in the Other Procedures section

Character 1	Character 2	Character 3	Character 4	Character 5	Character 6	Character 7
Section	Body System	Root Operation	Body Region	Approach	Method	Qualifier

- **Character 6 (Method):** Defines the method of the procedure, such as robotic-assisted procedure, computer-assisted procedure, or acupuncture

Coding Note: Other Procedures Section
The Other Procedures section contains codes for procedures not included in the other Medical and Surgical-related sections. There are relatively few procedures coded in this section. Whole body therapies including acupuncture and meditation are included in this section along with a code for the fertilization portion of an in-vitro fertilization procedure. This section also contains codes for robotic-assisted and computer-assisted procedures.

Root Operation

Other Procedures: 0

Definition   Methodologies that attempt to remediate or cure a disorder or disease

Explanation For nontraditional whole-body therapies including acupuncture and meditation

Example Acupuncture

Additional Examples of Other Procedures

- Robotic-assisted transurethral prostatectomy
- Suture removal, abdominal wall
- Computer-assisted coronary artery bypass
- Robotic-assisted hysterectomy
- Yoga therapy
- CT computer-assisted sinus surgery
- Near infrared spectroscopy of leg vessels

Chiropractic: 9

The seven characters in the Chiropractic section are shown in figure 11.9.

Figure 11.9. The seven characters in the Chiropractic section are:

Character 1	Character 2	Character 3	Character 4	Character 5	Character 6	Character 7
Section	Body System	Root Operation	Body Region	Approach	Method	Qualifier

- **Character 2 (Body System):** Single body system value, **Anatomical Regions**

Coding Note: Chiropractic Section
Section 9, Chiropractic, consists of a single body system, Anatomical Regions, and a single root operation, Manipulation

Root Operation

Manipulation: B

Definition Manual procedures that involve a direct thrust to move a joint past the physiological range of motion, without exceeding the anatomical limit

Explanation None

Example   Chiropractic treatment of cervical spine, short
              lever specific contact

Additional Examples of Chiropractic Procedures

- Chiropractic treatment of lumbar region using long lever
  specific contact
- Chiropractic manipulation of abdominal region, indirect
  visceral
- Chiropractic extra-articular treatment of left hip region
- Chiropractic treatment of sacrum using long and short lever
  specific contact
- Mechanically assisted chiropractic manipulation of head

Apply Knowledge to Transition from Coding in ICD-9-CM to ICD-10-PCS

Case Example #1

The following case is for a dilation and curettage following an incomplete spontaneous abortion which is coded to 69.02 in ICD-9-CM. The code descriptor for 69.02 is Dilation and curettage following delivery and abortion and is categorized under category 69, Other operations on uterus and supporting structures. A coding professional would code 69.02 whether or not the procedure was performed with or without a scope. If an aspiration curettage had been performed, the correct code would be 69.52, not 69.02.

Case Description: The patient is a 25-year-old female, gravida 2, para 1, in her tenth week of pregnancy. While at work, she developed severe cramping and vaginal bleeding. Co-workers brought her to the hospital emergency room, and she was admitted to the hospital. After examination, the physician described her condition as an "inevitable abortion." The physician subsequently documented that the patient had an incomplete early spontaneous abortion. During this pregnancy the patient had been treated for transient hypertension of pregnancy, for which she was monitored during this hospital stay. She was taken to the operating room where a dilation and curettage was performed to treat the abortion. There were no complications from the procedure and the patient was subsequently discharged.

Case Explanation: A dilation and curettage following an incomplete spontaneous abortion is coded to the root operation Extraction (10**D**17ZZ) in the Obstetrics section of ICD-10-PCS. This procedure is coded to the Obstetrics section since the procedure was performed on the products of conception. ICD-10-PCS coding guideline C2 states that "procedures performed following a delivery or abortion for curettage of the endometrium or evacuation of retained products of conception are coded in the Obstetrics section, to the root operation Extraction and the body part Products of Conception, Retained". ICD-10-PCS does not differentiate between a dilation and curettage and aspiration curettage. Therefore 10D17ZZ would be coded for both of these procedures.

Case Example #2

A coding professional would code this case to 74.1 in ICD-9-CM. The code descriptor for 74.1 is Low cervical cesarean section and is categorized to category 74, Cesarean section and removal of fetus. ICD-9-CM distinguishes the various types of cesarean sections at the third digit level.

Case Description: A 34-year-old female is admitted in active labor during week 39 of her pregnancy. She had a previous cesarean section two years previously as a result of fetal distress and cephalopelvic disproportion. No fetal distress was noted during this admission, but it was determined that the patient still had cephalopelvic disproportion; therefore, a repeat low cervical cesarean section was performed. A healthy 8 lb. 10 oz. female was delivered.

Case Explanation: The correct root operation for a cesarean section is Extraction (10**D**00Z1) as the objective of this procedure is to pull out the fetus (products of conception). Similar to ICD-9-CM, ICD-10-PCS differentiates the various types of cesarean sections. The seventh character of the ICD-10-PCS code captures the type of cesarean section.

Case Example #3

In ICD-9-CM a manually assisted vaginal delivery codes to 73.59, Other manually assisted delivery. Code 73.59 is categorized to category 73, Other procedures inducing or assisting delivery. There is only one

ICD-9-CM code for this procedure therefore all manually assisted deliveries are coded to 73.59.

Case Description: A 45-year-old woman, gravida 1, para 0, was admitted in labor to the hospital obstetrical department. The patient had been under the care of a physician who specialized in high-risk pregnancies. Because of her age, the woman was thought to be at higher risk for complications, but her pregnancy was uneventful. The physician described her as an "elderly primigravida, full term pregnancy." She had a manually assisted vaginal delivery of a healthy 7 lb. 5 oz. girl.

Case Explanation: Manually assisted deliveries code to the root operation Delivery (10E0XZZ) in ICD-10-PCS. The definition for Delivery is assisting the passage of the products of conception from the genital canal. Similar to ICD-9-CM, ICD-10-PCS has only one code for this procedure.

Case Example #4

The following case is the application of a cast on the right lower leg which is coded to 93.53 in ICD-9-CM. The code descriptor for 93.53 is Application of other cast and is categorized to category 93, Physical therapy, respiratory therapy, rehabilitation, and related procedures. ICD-9-CM does not differentiate the various body area or regions that a cast can be placed with twenty-eight different body areas or regions being coded to this code.

Case Description: The patient is a 67-year-old man who was seen in the office yesterday for a regular follow-up appointment for the management of his type 2 diabetes and his insulin dosage. The Accu-Chek performed in the office showed a result of 315. The patient stated his glucose is usually over 300 when he checks it at home. He reported feeling fairly well with a little more fatigue than usual. The patient is a retired truck driver and is fairly active, including helping his neighbors with yard work and snow shoveling. The patient is also known to have hypertension and chronic renal insufficiency that is fairly well controlled on medication. The patient was admitted to the hospital for control of his uncontrolled type 2 diabetes. The patient's 70/30 insulin was discontinued as well as the glyburide and Prandin. He was given Lantus insulin once a day with NovoLog with every meal. The patient was directed to monitor his glucose with every meal.

No other complications of his diabetes were found. His renal function was examined, and he was continued on his hypertensive medications. The patient also complained of pain in his right ankle that he said he sprained when he slipped while cleaning the snow off his car yesterday. An x-ray revealed a nondisplaced fracture of the lateral malleolus. An orthopedic consultation was obtained, and the patient was placed in a lower leg cast. No fracture reduction was required. Acquired spondylolisthesis of the ankle was also diagnosed. The patient will be seen in the primary care physician's office in 1 week and in the orthopedic surgeon's office in 4 weeks.

Case Explanation: The application of a cast to the right lower leg would code to the root operation Immobilization (2W3QX2Z) in ICD-10-PCS. Immobilization is limiting or preventing motion of a body region. This code is specifically for a cast application of only the right lower leg. Unlike ICD-9-CM, ICD-10-PCS provides distinct codes identifying the specific body area or region, including laterality, where the cast is being placed. The body area or region is captured with the fourth character of the ICD-10-PCS code.

Case Example #5

The following case is the application of a short arm splint to the left arm which is coded to 93.54 in ICD-9-CM. The code descriptor for 93.54 is Application of splint and is categorized to category 93, Physical therapy, respiratory therapy, rehabilitation, and related procedures. ICD-9-CM only provides one code for application of splint; therefore, all splint applications, except periodontal splint, code to 93.54.

Case Description: The patient is a 58-year-old male admitted with exacerbation of CHF. The patient also has hypertension and hypercholesterolemia which were managed throughout the hospital stay. On day 2 of the admission the patient mentioned that his left wrist has been bothering him for the past week or so. About a week ago the patient accidently tripped over his cat and fell to the floor striking his left wrist. An x-ray of the left wrist revealed a nondisplaced fracture of the radius. An orthopedic consultation was obtained, and the patient was placed in a short arm splint. The patient will be seen in the orthopedic physician's office in 2 weeks.

Case Explanation: The root operation for this procedure is Immobilization (2W3DX1Z) as the objective of this procedure is to limit or prevent the motion of the left lower arm. This code is specifically for a splint application of only the left lower arm. Unlike ICD-9-CM, ICD-10-PCS provides distinct codes identifying the specific body area or region, including laterality, where the splint is being placed. The body area or region is captured with the fourth character of the ICD-10-PCS code.

Case Example #6

In ICD-9-CM anterior nasal packing codes to 21.01, Control of epistaxis by anterior nasal packing. Code 21.01 is categorized to category 21, Operations on nose. ICD-9-CM provides distinct codes for the different types of nasal packing with 21.02 being used for both posterior nasal packing and anterior and posterior nasal packing. The code descriptor for 21.02 is Control of epistaxis by posterior (and anterior) packing

Case Description: The patient is a 46-year-old female who is being admitted for IV antibiotics to treat her urinary tract infection. A urine culture was done which revealed E. coli as the organism responsible for the UTI. On day 3 of the hospital stay the patient experienced some significant epistaxis which required anterior nasal packing.

Case Explanation: The root operation Packing (2Y41X5Z) would be used by the coding professional to code this procedure. Packing is defined as putting material in a body region or orifice. ICD-10-PCS provides only one code for nasal packing and does not differentiate between anterior, posterior, and combined anterior and posterior nasal packing.

Case Example #7

In ICD-9-CM the administration of chemotherapy codes to 99.25 with a code descriptor of Injection or infusion of cancer chemotherapeutic substances and is categorized under category 99.2, Injection or infusion of other therapeutic or prophylactic substance. ICD-9-CM provides only one code for the administration of antineoplastic agents and does not differentiate how it is administered such as through a central vein or artery, peripheral vein or artery, or by other routes such as into the spinal canal or a joint.

Case Description: This patient was admitted for chemotherapy following a recent diagnosis of carcinoma of the lower outer quadrant of the right breast. The patient underwent a mastectomy 3 months ago and she has been receiving chemotherapy. The patient also had a central venous catheter placed in the superior vena cava. The port of this catheter is being used for the chemotherapy treatment. After the chemotherapy was administered, the patient developed severe nausea and vomiting. Medications were given for the nausea and vomiting and the patient was subsequently discharged.

Case Explanation: The administration of a chemotherapy drug codes to the root operation Introduction (3E04305) within the Administration section of ICD-10-PCS. During an Introduction procedure a therapeutic, diagnostic, nutritional, physiological, or prophylactic substance is administered or put into the patient. Unlike ICD-9-CM, ICD-10-PCS differentiates the administration route which is captured with the fourth character of the code. Therefore, in ICD-10-PCS the code specifies whether the substance was administered via central vein or artery, peripheral vein or artery, or by other routes such as into the spinal canal or a joint.

Case Example #8

The following case is for a combined right and left heart catheterization which is coded to 37.23 in ICD-9-CM. The code descriptor for 37.23 is Combined right and left heart cardiac catheterization and is categorized in category 37, Other operations on heart and pericardium. ICD-9-CM differentiates between left heart catheterization, 37.22, right heart catheterization, 37.21, and combined heart catheterization, 37.23. Although a heart catheterization is usually performed percutaneously, occasionally the procedure is performed with an open approach. The code 37.23 is coded for both open and percutaneous combined right and left heart catheterizations.

Case Description: A 60-year-old male patient was admitted to the hospital with stable angina, which continued under treatment. He underwent a combined right and left heart cardiac catheterization with coronary angiography, Judkins technique, and was determined to have significant atherosclerotic heart disease. Triple coronary artery bypass surgery was recommended for the 70% to 80% occlusion found in three native coronary vessels. The patient was also treated for type 2 diabetes that has been well controlled. The patient requested that the open heart surgery be scheduled for a later date. The patient was subsequently discharged and will be scheduled for open heart surgery in 2 weeks. (**Note:** only comparing the codes for the left and right heart catheterization)

Case Explanation: A cardiac catheterization is coded to the root operation Measurement (4A023N8) in ICD-10-PCS. The root operation Measurement is used when the procedure is determining the level of physiological or physical function at a point in time. During a cardiac catheterization, measurements of pressures within the heart chamber(s) are taken. ICD-10-PCS differentiates the various approaches to performing this procedure with the fifth character capturing the approach.

Case Example #9

The following case is for an insertion of an endotracheal tube with subsequent mechanical ventilation for 36 hours which requires two codes. The insertion of the endotracheal tube codes to 96.04 in ICD-9-CM. The code descriptor for 96.04 is Insertion of an endotracheal tube and is categorized to category 96, Nonoperative intubation and irrigation. The mechanical ventilation is coded to 96.71 and has a code descriptor of Continuous invasive mechanical ventilation for less than 96 consecutive hours. ICD-9-CM provides three different codes for mechanical ventilation based on the number of consecutive hours: 96.70, unspecified duration, 96.71, for less than 96 consecutive hours, and 96.72, for 96 consecutive hours or more.

Case Description: The patient is a 65-year-old man with stage IV gastroesophageal junction carcinoma. He developed severe respiratory distress and was brought to the hospital emergency department and admitted. His condition progressed to acute respiratory failure, and he required intubation and mechanical ventilation for 36 hours.

Case Explanation: The root operation for the insertion of the endotracheal tube is Insertion (0BH17EZ) from the Medical and Surgical section of ICD-10-PCS. Insertion is defined as putting in a nonbiological appliance that monitors, assists, performs, or prevents a physiological function but does not physically take the place of the body part. The mechanical ventilation is coded to the root operation Performance in the Extracorporeal Assistance and Performance section (5A1945Z) of

ICD-10-PCS. Performance is defined as completely taking over a physiological function by extracorporeal means. In this case the mechanical ventilator is completely taking over the respiratory function. The range of consecutive hours for mechanical ventilation in ICD-10-PCS is different than ICD-9-CM. The ranges are less than 24 hours, 24–96 hours, or greater than 96 hours. Similar to ICD-9-CM, two codes are required to code this procedure.

Case Example #10

The following case is for a CABG × 4 with cardiopulmonary bypass which requires two codes. The CABG × 4 codes to 36.14 in ICD-9-CM. The code descriptor for 36.14 is Aortocoronary bypass of four or more coronary arteries and is categorized under category 36, Operations on vessels of heart. ICD-9-CM does not differentiate the type of graft material; therefore, 36.14 is coded for autologous venous tissue, autologous arterial tissue, synthetic substitute material, and nonautologous tissue substitute material.

The cardiopulmonary bypass codes to 39.61, Extracorporeal circulation auxiliary to open heart surgery. Code 39.61 is categorized to category 39, Other operations on vessels.

Case Description: A patient with severe arteriosclerotic heart disease of native arteries and severe chronic obstructive pulmonary disease was admitted for coronary artery bypass graft (CABG) × 4 with cardiopulmonary bypass. During the operative procedure all four coronary arteries were bypassed via the aortocoronary bypass technique utilizing saphenous vein grafts which had been harvested previously.

Case Explanation: The root operation for the CABG × 4 is Bypass (02**1**309W) from the Medical and Surgical section of ICD-10-PCS. ICD-10-PCS does differentiate the type of graft material being used with the sixth character of the code identifying the type of graft material. The root operation for the cardiopulmonary bypass is Performance (5A**1**221Z and 5A**1**935Z) from the Extracorporeal Assistance and Performance section of ICD-10-PCS. During cardiopulmonary bypass, the heart and lung machine is completely taking over two physiological functions, cardiac and respiratory; therefore, two codes are required.

Chapter 12

Ancillary Section

Definitions, Descriptions, and Examples of Root Types

ICD-10-PCS contains a total of six ancillary sections as shown in table 12.1.

Table 12.1. The six Ancillary sections of ICD-10-PCS

Section Value	Description
Section B	Imaging
Section C	Nuclear Medicine
Section D	Radiation Oncology
Section F	Physical Rehabilitation and Diagnostic Audiology
Section G	Mental Health
Section H	Substance Abuse Treatment

Note: Ancillary sections (sections B–D and F–H) do not include Root Operations. Character 3 represents Root Type of the procedure for these sections.

Imaging: B

The seven characters in the Imaging section are shown in figure 12.1.

Figure 12.1. The seven characters in the Imaging section

Character 1	Character 2	Character 3	Character 4	Character 5	Character 6	Character 7
Section	Body System	Root Type	Body Part	Contrast	Qualifier	Qualifier

Imaging follows the same conventions as the Medical and Surgical Section for the section (1), body system (2), and body part (4) characters. Characters 3, 5, 6, and 7 in the Imaging section are:

- **Character 3 (Root Type):** Defines procedure by root type, instead of root operation
- **Character 5 (Contrast):** Defines contrast if used; contrast is differentiated by the concentration of the contrast material (for example, high or low osmolar)
- **Character 6 (Qualifier):** Qualifier that specifies an image is taken without contrast followed by one with contrast (unenhanced and enhanced), or laser or intravascular optical coherence.
- **Character 7 (Qualifier):** Qualifier that has limited use in this section, but a few options are available (intraoperative, densitometry, or intravascular). When this qualifier is not applicable, the default value will be "Z."

Root Types

There are five Imaging root types as shown in table 12.2.

Table 12.2.   The five Imaging Root Types

Value	Description	Definition
0	Plain Radiography	Planar display of an image developed from the capture of external ionizing radiation on photographic or photoconductive plate
1	Fluoroscopy	Single plane or bi-plane real time display of an image developed from the capture of external ionizing radiation on a fluorescent screen. The image may also be stored by either digital or analog means
2	CT scan	Computer reformatted digital display of multiplanar images developed from the capture of multiple exposures of external ionizing radiation
3	Magnetic Resonance Imaging (MRI)	Computer reformatted digital display of multiplanar images developed from the capture of radio-frequency signals emitted by nuclei in a body site excited within a magnetic field
4	Ultrasonography	Real time display of images of anatomy or flow information developed from the capture of reflected and attenuated high frequency sound waves

Examples of Imaging Procedures

- Limited study x-ray of clavicle
- Chest x-ray, AP/PA and lateral views
- Portable x-ray study radius/ulna shaft, standard series
- Fluoroscopy of renal dialysis shunt
- Fluoroscopic guidance for percutaneous transluminal angio-plasty (PTA) of left common femoral artery, low osmolar contrast
- Esophageal videofluoroscopy study with oral barium contrast
- CT of brain without contrast followed by high osmolar contrast
- Non-contrast CT abdomen and pelvis
- CT scan bilateral lungs, high osmolar contrast with densitometry
- MRI liver
- MRI thyroid gland, unspecified contrast
- Ultrasound prostate
- Intravascular ultrasound subclavian artery
- Endoluminal ultrasound gallbladder and bile ducts
- Routine fetal ultrasound, second trimester twin gestation

Nuclear Medicine: C

The seven characters in the Nuclear Medicine section are shown in figure 12.2.

Figure 12.2.   The seven characters in the Nuclear Medicine section

Character 1	Character 2	Character 3	Character 4	Character 5	Character 6	Character 7
Section	Body System	Root Type	Body Part	Radionuclide	Qualifier	Qualifier

The characters that are of interest in the Nuclear Medicine section are:

- **Character 3 (Root Type):** Defines procedure by root type, instead of root operation
- **Character 5 (Radionuclide):** Defines the source of the radiation used in the procedure
- **Characters 6 and 7 (Qualifiers):** Are not specified in this section (Z)

Root Types

The root types in Nuclear Medicine are shown in table 12.3.

Table 12.3.   The seven Root Types in Nuclear Medicine

Value	Description	Definition
1	Planar Nuclear Medicine Imaging	Introduction of radioactive materials into the body for single plane display of images developed from the capture of radioactive emissions
2	Tomographic (Tomo) Nuclear Medicine Imaging	Introduction of radioactive materials into the body for three-dimensional display of images developed from the capture of radioactive emissions
3	Positron Emission Tomography (PET)	Introduction of radioactive materials into the body for three-dimensional display of images developed from the simultaneous capture, 180 degrees apart, of radioactive emissions
4	Nonimaging Nuclear Medicine Uptake	Introduction of radioactive materials into the body for measurements of organ function, from the detection of radioactive emissions
5	Nonimaging Nuclear Medicine Probe	Introduction of radioactive materials into the body for the study of distribution and fate of certain substances by the detection of radioactive emissions from an external source
6	Nonimaging Nuclear Medicine Assay	Introduction of radioactive materials into the body for the study of body fluids and blood elements, by the detection of radioactive emissions
7	Systemic Nuclear Medicine Therapy	Introduction of unsealed radioactive materials into the body for treatment

Examples of Nuclear Medicine Procedures

- Adenosine sestamibi (technetium) planar scan of heart muscle at rest
- Uniplanar scan of spine using technetium oxidronate, first pass study
- Gallium citrate scan head and neck, single plane imaging
- Upper GI scan, unspecified radiopharmaceutical for gastric emptying

- Technetium Tomo scan of liver
- Tomo scan right and left heart, qualitative gated rest
- Thallous chloride tomographic scan bilateral breasts
- PET scan myocardium using rubidium
- Carbon 11 PET scan brain with quantification
- Xenon gas nonimaging probe of brain
- Iodinated albumin nuclear medicine assay, blood plasma volume study
- Technetium pentetate assay kidneys, ureters, and bladder

Radiation Oncology: D

The seven characters in the Radiation Oncology section are shown in figure 12.3.

Figure 12.3. The seven characters in the Radiation Oncology section

Character 1	Character 2	Character 3	Character 4	Character 5	Character 6	Character 7
Section	Body System	Root Type	Treatment Site	Modality Qualifier	Isotope	Qualifier

- **Character 3 (Root Type):** Specifies the basic mode of radiation delivery used (beam radiation, brachytherapy, stereotactic radiosurgery, and other radiation)
- **Character 4 (Treatment Site):** Specifies the body part that is the target of the radiation therapy
- **Character 5 (Modality Qualifier):** Further specifies the type of radiation used (photons, electrons, heavy particles, contact radiation)
- **Character 6 (Isotope):** Specifies the isotope administered in the oncology treatment
- **Character 7 (Qualifier):** Allows for the reporting of intraoperative procedures. If not applicable, the "Z" is assigned.

Root Types

The third character root types are shown in table 12.4.

Table 12.4.   The third character Root Types

Value	Description
0	Beam Radiation
1	Brachytherapy
2	Stereotactic Radiosurgery
Y	Other Radiation

Examples of Radiation Oncology Procedures

- 8 MeV photon beam radiation to brain
- Heavy particle radiation treatment pancreas, four risk sites
- Electron radiation treatment breast, custom device
- LDR (low dose rate) brachytherapy of cervix using Iridium 192
- HDR (high dose rate) brachytherapy prostate using Palladium 103
- LDR brachytherapy spinal cord using iodine
- Intraoperative radiation therapy (IORT) of bladder
- Plaque radiation eye, single port
- IORT intraoperative radiation therapy colon, 3 ports
- Hyperthermia oncology treatment pelvic region
- Contact radiation tongue

Physical Rehabilitation and Diagnostic Audiology: F

The seven characters in the Physical Rehabilitation and Diagnostic Audiology section are shown in figure 12.4.

Figure 12.4.   The seven characters in the Physical Rehabilitation and Diagnostic Audiology section

Character 1	Character 2	Character 3	Character 4	Character 5	Character 6	Character 7
Section	Section Qualifier	Root Type	Body System/ Region	Type Qualifier	Equipment	Qualifier

- **Character 2 (Section Qualifier):** Specifies whether the procedure is a rehabilitation or diagnostic audiology procedure
- **Character 3 (Root Type):** Specifies general procedure root type

- **Character 4 (Body System/Region):** Specifies the body system and body region combined, where applicable
- **Character 5 (Type Qualifier):** Specifies the precise test or method employed. These are well defined in the system. An example is for root type Activities of daily living treatment, fifth character value of 0 is for bathing/showering techniques.
- **Character 6 (Equipment):** Specifies the general categories of equipment used, if any (note: specific types of equipment are not listed)
- **Character 7 (Qualifier):** Not specified in this section

Root Types

The Physical Rehabilitation and Diagnostic Audiology section classifies procedures into the 14 root types shown in table 12.5.

Table 12.5.   The 14 Root Types in the Physical Rehabilitation and Diagnostic Audiology section

Value	Description	Definition
0	Speech Assessment	Measurement of speech and related functions
1	Motor and/or Nerve Function Assessment	Measurement of motor, nerve, and related functions
2	Activities of Daily Living Assessment	Measurement of functional level for activities of daily living
3	Hearing Assessment	Measurement of hearing and related functions
4	Hearing Aid Assessment	Measurement of the appropriateness and/or effectiveness of a hearing device
5	Vestibular Assessment	Measurement of the vestibular system and related functions
6	Speech Treatment	Application of techniques to improve, augment, or compensate for speech and related functional impairment
7	Motor Treatment	Exercise or activities to increase or facilitate motor function
8	Activities of Daily Living Treatment	Exercise or activities to facilitate functional competence for activities of daily living
9	Hearing Treatment	Application of techniques to improve, augment, or compensate for hearing and related functional impairment

(Continued on next page)

Table 12.5.   (Continued)

Value	Description	Definition
B	Hearing Aid Treatment	Application of techniques to improve the communication abilities of individuals with cochlear implant
C	Vestibular Treatment	Application of techniques to improve, augment, or compensate for vestibular and related functional impairment
D	Device Fitting	Fitting of a device designed to facilitate or support achievement of a higher level of function. **NOTE**: Device Fitting describes the device being fitted rather than the method used to fit the device.
F	Caregiver Training	Training in activities to support patient's optimal level of function. **NOTE:** Caregiver Training is divided into 18 different broad subjects taught to help a caregiver provide proper patient care.

Coding Note: Treatment
Treatment procedures include swallowing dysfunction exercises, bathing and showering techniques, wound management, gait training, and a host of activities typically associated with rehabilitation.

Coding Note: Assessment
Assessments are further classified into more than 100 different tests or methods. The majority of these focus on the faculties of hearing and speech, but others focus on various aspects of body function, and on the patient's quality of life, such as muscle performance, neuromotor development, and reintegration skills.

Examples of Physical Rehabilitation and Diagnostic Audiology Procedures

- Wound care treatment calf ulcer using pulsatile lavage
- Articulation and phonology assessment using spectrograph
- Individual fitting moveable knee brace
- Caregiver training in feeding

- Bekesy assessment using audiometer
- Individual fitting eye prosthesis
- Physical therapy for range of motion and mobility of hip
- Bedside swallow assessment
- Caregiver training in airway clearance techniques
- Application short arm cast in rehab
- Verbal assessment patient's pain level
- Caregiver training in communication skills using manual communication board
- Group musculoskeletal balance training exercises, whole body
- Individual therapy for auditory processing using tape recorder

Mental Health Section: G

The seven characters in the Mental Health section are shown in figure 12.5.

Figure 12.5.   The seven characters in the Mental Health section

Character 1	Character 2	Character 3	Character 4	Character 5	Character 6	Character 7
Section	Body System	Root Type	Type Qualifier	Qualifier	Qualifier	Qualifier

- **Character 2 (Body System):** Does not convey specific information about the procedure; the value Z functions as a placeholder for this character
- **Character 3 (Root Type):** Specifies the mental health procedure root type
- **Character 4 (Type Qualifier):** Further specifies the procedure type as needed
- **Characters 5, 6, and 7 (Qualifier):** Do not convey specific information about the procedure, the value Z functions as a placeholder for these characters

Root Types

The Mental Health section classifies procedures into the 11 Root Types shown in table 12.6.

Table 12.6.   The 11 Root Types in the Mental Health section

Value	Description
1	Psychological Tests
2	Crisis Intervention
5	Individual Psychotherapy
6	Counseling
7	Family Psychotherapy
B	Electroconvulsive Therapy
C	Biofeedback
F	Hypnosis
G	Narcosynthesis
H	Group Therapy
J	Light Therapy

Examples of Mental Health Procedures

- Galvanic skin response (GSR) biofeedback
- Cognitive-behavioral individual psychotherapy
- Narcosynthesis
- Light therapy
- Electroconvulsive therapy (ECT), unilateral, multiple seizure
- Crisis intervention
- Neuropsychological testing
- Hypnosis
- Developmental testing
- Vocational counseling
- Family psychotherapy

Substance Abuse Treatment: H

The seven characters in the Substance Abuse Treatment section are shown in figure 12.6.

Figure 12.6. **The seven characters in the Substance Abuse Treatment section**

Character 1	Character 2	Character 3	Character 4	Character 5	Character 6	Character 7
Section	Body System	Root Type	Type Qualifier	Qualifier	Qualifier	Qualifier

- **Character 2 (Body System):** Does not convey specific information about the procedure, the value Z functions as a placeholder for this character
- **Character 3 (Root Type):** Specifies the root type
- **Character 4 (Type Qualifier):** Further classifies the root type
- **Characters 5, 6, and 7 (Qualifier):** Do not convey specific information about the procedure, the value Z functions as a placeholder for these characters

Root Types

The seven different root type values in the Substance Abuse Treatment section are shown in table 12.7.

Table 12.7. **The seven Root Types in the Substance Abuse Treatment section**

Value	Description
2	Detoxification Services
3	Individual Counseling
4	Group Counseling
5	Individual Psychotherapy
6	Family Counseling
8	Medication Management
9	Pharmacotherapy

Examples of Substance Abuse Treatment

- Pharmacotherapy treatment with Antabuse for alcohol addiction
- Naltrexone treatment for drug dependency

- Substance abuse treatment family counseling
- Medication monitoring of patient on methadone maintenance
- Individual interpersonal psychotherapy for drug abuse
- Patient for alcohol detoxification treatment
- Group motivational counseling
- Individual 12-step psychotherapy for substance abuse
- Post-test infectious disease counseling for IV drug abuser
- Psychodynamic psychotherapy for drug dependent patient
- Group cognitive-behavioral counseling for substance abuse

Apply Knowledge to Transition from Coding in ICD-9-CM to ICD-10-PCS

Case Example #1

The following case is for an operative cholangiography done prior to a Roux-en-Y cholecystojejunostomy of the gallbladder. The intraoperative cholangiography is coded to 87.53 in ICD-9-CM. The code descriptor for 87.53 is Intraoperative cholangiogram and is categorized under category 87.5, Biliary tract x-ray. The principal procedure, the Roux-en-Y cholecystojejunostomy is coded 51.32. The code descriptor for 51.32 is Anastomosis of gallbladder to intestine and is categorized under category 51.3, Anastomosis of gallbladder or bile duct

Case Description: A 3-month-old infant is born with a biliary atresia. The patient has severe obstructive jaundice due to the congenital condition. The patient was admitted and the diagnosis is confirmed by surgical exploration with operative cholangiography. The biliary atresia is treated with laparoscopic Roux-en-Y cholecystojejunostomy of the gallbladder.

Case Explanation: To correctly code the cholangiogram, it is helpful to understand something about the procedure. Typically the procedure is performed to identify structures during other biliary tract surgery. The cystic duct at the gallbladder neck is identified, and a small ductotomy made. Then a cholangio catheter is threaded and radiographic contrast is infused through the catheter and fluoroscopic images are obtained of the biliary system. In this particular procedure, the section in ICD-10-PCS is Imaging (B) and the body system is Hepatobiliary System and Pancreas (F). To determine the root type, documentation should indicate if fluoroscopy was used or not, since in ICD-10-PCS the Index provides

Cholangiogram
  See Plain Radiography, Hepatobiliary System and Pancreas BF0
  See Fluoroscopy, Hepatobiliary System and Pancreas BF1

Once documentation is reviewed to determine the root type, the specific body part must be determined. Depending on the root type, body parts might be: Bile ducts; Gallbladder and bile ducts; Hepatobiliary system: all; Biliary and pancreatic ducts; Gallbladder; Gallbladder, bile ducts and pancreatic ducts; or pancreatic ducts. After the specific body part(s) are determined one must know what type of contrast media is used (high osmolar, low osmolar, or other contrast). It is evident that the ICD-10-PCS code is much more specific than the ICD-9-CM code. Based on the limited documentation provided (that which would have easily produced an ICD-9-CM code) more specific documentation is need to assign this code in ICD-10-PCS.

To code the Roux-en-Y cholecystojejunostomy procedure, the root operation is bypass, with the body system of hepatobiliary system and pancreas (0F144ZB). A cholecystojejunostomy is an anastomosis of the gallbladder and the jejunum. In ICD-10-PCS, the code for the body part (gallbladder) (character 4) is the origin of the bypass, and the qualifier (character 7) (jejunum) identifies the destination of the bypass.

Case Example #2

The following case is for supportive verbal psychotherapy coded to 94.38 in ICD-9-CM. The code descriptor for 94.38 is Supportive verbal psychotherapy and is categorized under category 94.3, Individual psychotherapy.

Case Description: A patient with bipolar disorder, type II, most recently in a depressed state, was admitted to the hospital with side effects due to the prescription lithium carbonate she had been taking. According to her caregivers, the drug had been administered correctly, and there was no possibility of a drug overdose. The patient had been sleeping 20 hours a day and was diagnosed with a drug-induced hypersomnia as a result of lithium toxicity. A therapeutic drug level for the lithium carbonate was found to be increased. The dosage was adjusted, and the patient received individual supportive verbal psychotherapy for the bipolar disorder while in the hospital. The patient was able to be discharged to the residential living center where she resided.

Case Explanation: This mental health procedure codes to the root type of individual psychotherapy (GZ**5**6ZZZ) in ICD-10-PCS. The fourth character (6) specifies that it is supportive therapy. In ICD-10-PCS there is also a series of codes for individual psychotherapy when done for substance abuse (HZ5).

Case Example #3

The following case is for detoxification for drug abuse which is coded to 94.65 in ICD-9-CM. The code descriptor for 94.65 is Drug detoxification and is categorized under category 94.6, Alcohol and drug rehabilitation and detoxification.

Case Description: After numerous drug possession arrests, a 40-year-old man was mandated to the substance abuse treatment facility for admission to undergo detoxification for his continuous cocaine addiction.

Case Explanation: The drug detoxification procedure in the Substance Abuse Section (H) would code to the root type Detoxification Services (HZ**2**ZZZZ). This code is the only choice for detoxification services, and includes alcohol and/or drugs. If substance abuse counseling or other treatment was performed, it would also be coded based upon the specific type of therapy (individual counseling, group counseling, individual psychotherapy, family counseling, medication management, or pharmacotherapy).

Resources

Centers for Medicare & Medicaid Services. 2010. 2010 Code Tables and Index. http://www.cms.hhs.gov/ICD10.

Centers for Medicare & Medicaid Services. 2009. ICD-10 Overview. http://www.cms.gov/ICD10/.

Centers for Medicare & Medicaid Services. 2010. ICD-10-PCS Reference Manual and Slides; Development of the ICD-10 Procedure Coding System (ICD-10-PCS); and 2011 Official ICD-10-PCS Coding Guidelines. http://www.cms.hhs.gov/ICD10.

Dorland. 2003. *Dorland's Illustrated Medical Dictionary*. Philadelphia, PA: W.B. Saunders.

Department of Health and Human Services. n.d. http://www.nhlbi.nih.gov/health/dci/Diseases/hhw/hhw_anatomy.html.

Encyclopedia Britannica. 2009. Human reproductive system. http://www.britannica.com/EBchecked/topic/498625/human-reproductive-system.

National Cancer Institute. n.d. http://training.seer.cancer.gov/.

National Heart Lung and Blood Institute. n.d. http://www.nhlbi.nih.gov/health/dci/Diseases/Angioplasty/Angioplasty_howdone.html.

National Institutes of Health. National Heart Lung and Blood Institute. Disease and Conditions Index. http://www.nhlbi.nih.gov/health/dci/index.html.

National Library of Medicine. n.d. http://gateway.nlm.nih.gov/gw/Cmd?GMMTSearch%26loc=nccs.